# TRUTH GAMES

# Truth Games

## Lies, Money, and Psychoanalysis

JOHN FORRESTER

HARVARD UNIVERSITY PRESS

Cambridge, Massachusetts
London, England
1997

*Library of Congress Cataloging-in-Publication Data*

Forrester, John.
Truth games : lies, money, and psychoanalysis /
John Forrester.
p.   cm.
Includes bibliographical references and index.
ISBN 0-674-53962-1 (alk. paper)
1. Psychoanalysis.   2. Psychoanalytic interpretation.
3. Freud, Sigmund, 1856–1939.   4. Lacan, Jacques, 1901–1981.   I. Title.
BF175.F655   1997
150.19′5—dc21       97-17559

*For Lisa,*
*who more than does*

# CONTENTS

# FOREWORD
## Adam Phillips

In obeying the fundamental rule of free association—what John Forrester calls in this book "the breathtakingly imperialistic requirement to reveal all"—the person entering analysis agrees to suspend, or at least to defer, the evaluation of what he says. The distinction between truth and lies is assumed to be a resistance to speaking freely, an obstacle rather than an instrument. Telling the truth in analysis, that is to say, means relinquishing one's wish to tell the truth. The patient has to stop weighing his words. The liar, after all, is the one who is supposed to know at least what the truth is; only knowledge of the truth would make one lie.

Speech becomes fuller, Freud discovered—more interestingly meaningful—if the analyst also abjures the criteria of truthfulness. It is as if with the concept of truth—and money: our currencies gain currency, as Forrester shows, by doubling for each other—we have been bewitched into believing that there is an ultimate, foolproof, universal object of desire, and that its legitimacy is beyond question. To ask what else we could want seems both silly and suspect. "Telling the truth," Forrester mentions, "never raises questions about one's motives, whereas telling lies always does." Good words make a good life; but psychoanalysis makes us wonder what good words are true to.

It was the figure Freud called the censor—originally the magistrate who kept accounts of the property of Roman citizens, imposed taxes, and watched over their morals—who appeared to know both what was worth saying, and to whom. Precursor of the superego, it was the function of the censor, who combined the severe moralism of the aesthete and the dutifulness of the customs official, to discriminate: between pleasure and pain, good and bad, truth and lies. All judgment, Freud implied, is punishing. All truth-claims are triumphalist.

In rather a stark sense psychoanalysis depends upon the censor; without the notion of censorship, the theoretical system is unintelligible. Without the possibility that the censorship itself can be censored—that it is subject to modification, that it can recognize an authority other than its own—psychoanalytic treatment is futile. From a psychoanalytic point of view censorship is the paradigmatic speech act, the need to render something acceptable. But if, as Forrester writes in this patient and startling book, "psychoanalysis always subordinates the discourse of blame to the discourse of discovery," how does it do something that is so against the grain of the moral imagination? What else can we do with the unacceptable but blame it for something? What, in other words, does psychoanalysis promise, what is the patient entitled to expect? In *Truth Games* Forrester shows us, among many other things, how psychoanalysis radically redescribes the twin notions of the promise and the contract: the foundations, dependent as they are on trust and good faith, of the erotic and of the marketplace. The psychoanalytic contract, he suggests, reveals both the ironic impossibility and the virtual necessity of contract. Children have to be sufficiently agreeable to their parents, but they don't make an agreement with them.

It is one of the paradoxes of beginning an analysis that the patient agrees to buy something that no one can really describe. Psychoanalysis has its history, its theory, its rules, and indeed those news bulletins called case histories. But what is going to be said and what is going to be heard—and the consequences of all that ritualized speaking and listening and silence—are forever beyond anticipation. What the analyst and the patient will make of each other is always an unknown quantity. In this sense psychoanalysis is both the exemplary and the parodic commodity: the kind of investment no rational person could possibly make. You pay money for an indefinite period to somebody you know very little about; this person, who doesn't say very much, has no idea what the return on your money will be, but knows it will be painful whatever else it is (from a psychoanalytic point of view, only what is unacceptable is, as it were, in a position to return). What your money allows you to give to the analyst is what you are able, or enabled, to say in her presence. And the words that she gives back to you serve to make more of your words possible, or valuable. But it is not words for words' sake; it is words to relieve suffering, to make something newly bearable. The analyst and the patient trade vocabularies to make a good difference, without knowing what the good will be. The analysis is bought on trust; the currency, as Forrester's title intimates, is truth games, lies, money, and Freud. But what exactly is on offer?

It has been one of the abiding preoccupations of Forrester's prolific, shrewdly informed work to describe the nature of the exchange that is psychoanalysis, and the histories of the institutionalized exchanges that are its precursors. In the two essays that make up this book—which should be read as two linked intellectual novellas, a Bildungsroman of ideas—Forrester addresses with a new kind of attention the really very strange, deadpan question posed in *The Seductions of Psychoanalysis:* "What is the story of the unconscious?" What are our stories about it—stories that inevitably interweave competing discourses—and what kinds of stories does "it" tell?

Psychoanalysis assumes that all stories, of whatever kind of coherence or intelligibility, are histories: histories of what we want, and of how our wanting works—and of the relationship, if any, between what we want from each other and what we can be said to give to each other (Lacan terminally ironized the gift, Forrester suggests, whereas Freud made of indebtedness a tragedy). What is distinctive about the histories Forrester has to tell in *Truth Games*—and history, Forrester has often implied, is the meeting point (or the melting point) between gossip and scholarship—is that they are, as it were, genealogies without piety and nostalgia. They situate psychoanalysis—in relation to epistemology (truth games), economic theory (gift, money, and debt), and the history of medicine (particularly the placebo effect and its link with hysteria)—without overcontextualizing it. There is no background for psychoanalysis to fade into, but there is some limelight for it to steal. What Forrester wants to claim, following from Nietzsche, is our need now, in the light of what he calls "the blithely truth-serving epistemologies of the natural sciences," for a psychopathology of the truthteller. And what Forrester wants more blithely to proclaim, following (agonistically) from Lacan—against, that is to say, the Symbolic as a synonym for the obsessionality of debt—is an acknowledgment that "our deepest wishes are for something that is as gratuitous, as full of grace, as happiness. The gift of something for nothing." Forrester, in other words (that are his) wants to keep psychoanalysis as a "pure culture of the life-instinct."

If the hero of the first essay is the child who lies, the hero of the second essay is the child whose desire is not for money. The child's first successful lie to the parents, Freud stated, was his first moment of independence (or freedom, to use the old-fashioned word). By making himself opaque to his parents, the child proves that the parents are not omniscient, not of the same mind as he. What is morally unacceptable—the lie—is developmentally essential. The child's capacity of lying, his talent for deception, guarantees his future (honesty is a symbiotic fantasy). But if children need to learn how to lie, they also have to learn to want money. What is most remarkable about *Truth Games* is the way in which Forrester has made and elaborated the connection between these two simple and apparently disparate things. "Infantile wishes are foreign to the logic of money," as Forrester says, but compatible with, if not integral to, the logic of dissimulation.

Quoting Freud's famous letter to Fliess—"Happiness is the belated fulfillment of a prehistoric wish. For this reason wealth brings so little happiness. Money was not a childhood wish"—Forrester, making one of the many telling connections that characterize this book, links

Freud's remarks to the fact that at the time of this letter—early in 1898—Freud was at last detaching himself from his fateful relationship with Breuer, by attempting to pay off his extensive financial debt to him. But paying off the money, of course, didn't cancel out the relationship (Freud went on guiltily and gratefully referring to Breuer until the early 1930s). There is, as Forrester notes, "no means of measuring symbolic debt"; by quantifying debt, money provides a spurious absolution. What we owe each other, like what links us to each other, is singularly lacking in definition (and, what do they amount to, our obligations and our relationships? seems like the wrong question, but the accounting still goes on). It is in the implications of indebtedness that Forrester finds his theme: in the no man's land between obligation and desire.

What does the child owe the parents: truth or lies, compliance or development? What does the child want from the parents, and how does he distinguish this from his obligation to them? Is speaking itself, to take Forrester's salient example, a repayment of the debt of language, a repayment of the words invested in us by our parents? In *Truth Games* Forrester circles these questions psychoanalytically: that is in the fullest sense, historically, not through the available reductions of child development, or the economic and ideological determinisms, but rather by interleaving a concise history of the genres of truth-telling with a sharp account of the evolution of economic systems.

When Lacan reads Freud it is as though, Forrester suggests, he is under some terrible obligation—as though in all his ironic exhilaration he is showing us how demanding the dead are. Lacan reminded us that on virtually every page of Freud there was a reference to language; Forrester points out that on virtually every page of Lacan there is no quotation from Freud. These are the strategies of transmission: ways of unburdening the past. *Truth Games* shows us how we can make a gift of our inheritance.

# INTRODUCTION

Everyday life contains many truth games. The social processes and institutions that establish power, expertise, and authority also generate truths. In deference to their formal structure and their internal rationality, but in a spirit of agnosticism concerning their claims, one against the other, to the Truth, we can call these procedures truth games.[1] We seek the truth through the courts, in scientific laboratories, in our religious institutions, and in private from those we love. Each of these processes gives rise to truths, more or less generally accepted but not necessarily compatible with one another. In large part, we accept the differences between them and, once we have been acclimatized, we know reasonably well the different rules, the different answers, the different prohibitions and failures of courtesy, taste, and etiquette proper to each.

Our own good behavior does not prevent us from enjoying the spectacle of transgression of the rules defining each of these games. This enjoyment often embodies the hope that a transcendent truth will, under the pressure of these transgressions, eventually break through, revealing something beyond the earthbound truths whose human failings and limitations we are, on those rare occasions when we want to be, only too well aware of. So, the spectacle of the scientist uncomfortably cornered by a terrier-like journalist, or a prelate confessing his sexual predilections over the dinner table, or a judge who reveals her ignorance of the latest fashion—whether it is a sophisticated new forensic laboratory technique or the name of a rock group—all of these give us a social delight arising out of the carnivalesque transgression of the rules of the game. We know full well that, in the morning, things will go back to normal: scientists will have an unquestioned authority over their specialized domains of expertise; priests will incarnate moral authority over matters public and private; judges will have dominion over matters of life and death, criminality and liberty. None of this prevents truth games from changing their rules, often more rapidly than we would like, and almost always without our agreement.

In the normal run of things, we take the plurality of truths for granted. We inhabit the games that generate them without any feeling of outlandishness or oddity. The fact that these games are often allied to an array of institutions, each with uncontested authority over truth claims made in its name—among them the law, medicine, the churches, the sciences, the central bank when allied with the arms-bearing state—does not strike us as perverse. It seems natural that banks should control money rather than pass judgment, and equally natural that being proficient at controlling money confers no authority over the conduct of surgery. However, it has been argued with great persuasiveness that this separation of institutional powers and authority is the distinctive and unusual feature of Western societies as they have developed in this millennium.[2] There might have been, there might still be, just one way of deciding a question as to truth, instead of the variety of ways which we live by and with. We certainly are only too aware of contests between rival institutions, between rival procedures. The warfare between science and religion was one; the rivalry between doctors and lawyers over unreasonable law-breaking actions was another; covert and not so covert tugs of war between politicians and their scientific advisers are becoming routine; and in the United States, the lawyers and the journalists increasingly vie for the highest public function of supreme adversary of those who would deny or cover up the truth, whether it be about killer viruses, arms scams, or athletic lovers.

We give the name "scientism" to the conviction that scientific truth should have hegemony over other truths, and that scientific institutions therefore have a privilege in relation to other institutions. We live in the age of scientism: by which I do not mean that scientism has been accepted, simply that ours is the age in which it is a continual presence, a continual seduction. One may be extremely sympathetic to its seductions, one may be extremely impressed by the successes of the sciences and their interdependent technologies, but that should not prevent us from recognizing how extremely vulnerable we are to scientism, nor from recognizing that its victory would spell the end of the distinctive plurality of truth games which constitutes the present dispensation for truth in our world.

What are the best ways of investigating this present dispensation of our truth games, including the insistent longing for the definitive scientific answer? When practitioners, institutions, whole discourses lay claim to their truths, the obvious point of entry into the foundations of their claims is the manner in which they exclude threats to the well-foundedness of those claims. The liar emerged for me as the exemplary figure of the outcast from those competing discourses. Error and ignorance, as the obverse of truth, appear as less interesting and threatening than lies. Each discourse or institution has its procedures for dealing with error and ignorance, which range from the legal fiction that ignorance is no defense to the philosopher's fiction that error, in the form of a bold but falsified hypothesis, is the highest scientific virtue. The liar, however, can become a truly subversive and scandalous figure, whose nefarious influence may extend far more widely than her own individual actions. Every truth-establishing institution has its own version of the liar: in the realm of economic transactions, there are the counterfeiter and fraudster; in the realm of politics, there are the Nixons, Hitlers, and Stalins—we even remain content with a definition of the diplomat as someone sent abroad to lie for his country; in the sciences, there are the Kammerers and Burts. But I had additional reasons for thinking that lying was a profitable area of inquiry.

Our century has given rise to a most original form of scientism: the quest for a science of the intimate and private person, a science of our moral inclinations, imperatives, failings, and hypocrisies—in short, a science of the individual life and of its fateful tragedies and comic fatalities. That project is psychoanalysis. It is well for us to recall the hopes and confidence that attended the rise and expansion of psychoanalysis—not least because we live at a moment when those most imbued with scientism repudiate as vociferously as the laws of libel and slander will allow the claims to scientific status of the somewhat becalmed flagship of their movement.[3] Part of the revolutionary, even flamboyant, promise of psychoanalysis was its pledge to reveal the underbelly of all other truths: of the physicist's truths, of the politician's, not to mention the more obviously targeted judge's and priest's truths. All that was necessary was for them to lie on the couch. Freud proposed that no area of discourse should be closed to the analyst's inquiry; and he also offered the rule of thumb that the sexual life of each individual should be considered as the model for his or her activity in all other areas of life, in the process proposing that sex be regarded as the ultimate truth about human beings.

However, allied with the breathtakingly imperialistic requirement to reveal all is the psychoanalyst's limitless tolerance for the subject's inability—his refusal—to speak the truth. Psychoanalysis is thus an intriguing example of a scientistic discourse that is focused on the intimate truths of everyday life, while redrawing the conventional lines between truth and lies. Might the psychoanalytic equanimity concerning lying offer a clue as to the manner in which other truth games, which are markedly less tolerant in this respect, regulate their practitioners and manage their relations with other, competing truth-seeking institutions? Could it be that the transgressions of truth and the truth game played by the psychoanalyst, that connoisseur of transgression, show us the means of discovering how we are governed by the various regimes of truth under which we now live? This book attempts to show that the answers that flow from this question are, at the very least, intriguing.

———

I have lived with the ideas in this book for a long time, long past the nine years enjoined by Horace. It was Lacan who first kindled my

interest in the topic of lying, with his observation that the psychoanalyst's patient is, even when lying, operating in the dimension of
truth. If such is the case, I reflected, then psychoanalysis must
operate with a very different notion of the rules connecting truth and
lies from those implied by the blacks and whites of the moral condemnation or the blithely truth-serving epistemologies of the natural
sciences. I also quickly came to recognize that the lies of childhood,
my own included, were, as philosophers, psychologists, and pedagogues insisted, of great significance. There are those who acquire
the habit of lying in a spectacular and dramatic manner, transforming
their lives in the process. For them, lying can have a foundationally
creative function; that first lie marks the opening of their own personal truths. But then there are those who have always lied, whose
lies as a consequence appear somewhat inconsequential, just a habit,
like playing with their hair. For these, lying was more a natural
disposition, akin to enthusiasm for sex or sport, than a matter of life
and death. My growing awareness of the interesting variety of lies
and of liars, fully sustained by numerous conversations and encounters in which I was told of the most horrendous, entertaining, and
extravagant bouts of lying, led me to realize that this was a topic
about which many people felt enthusiastic and perplexed. This recognition kept me working on the topic, on and off, over a period of
twenty years.

At some point in the work, about ten years ago, I became preoccupied with the questions of trust and confidence that are linked to
the endemic fear of lying. If the world were full of liars, the argument
so often ran, how could we trust what other people said? This
argument, it seemed to me, always put the cart before the horse. As
all people seem to agree when they are living in their unofficial
worlds, there is a great deal of hard lying that goes on in the world,
especially among those we most respect and admire. But, nonetheless,
we live in a world in which there is trust; how much lying goes on
in that world appears to be a matter for disinterested empirical
inquiry rather than philosophical anxiety, and may bear only very
indirectly on the basic attitude of trust. A venerable parallel began

5

to impress me, that between the trust underlying the institution of truth-saying and the trust underlying the institution of economic exchange. Counterfeiters are the liars of the economic world, and their attack on the institution of money seems very much akin to the liar's parasitic attack on the institution of truth. Are not both institutions dependent, as all the commentators seem to agree, on trust? And are not both institutions therefore always in need of something deeper, more solid, more foundational, more rocklike, than trust upon which to base that trust?

I explore the parallel between money and speech in the second essay in this book, through an examination of the metaphors of circulation, exchange, indebtedness, and trust that slide incessantly from one domain to the other, from words to coins and back again. The essay opens by looking at the relationship between Lacan and Freud, but it soon extends to the broader questions of the anthropology, the economics, and the metaphysics that underpin psychoanalysis and the human sciences. And it closes with the conclusion that the concepts which we find it impossible to relinquish when we assess human relations and human connectedness, the concepts of gift and debt, are irremediably unstable, riven with internal contradictions whose effects we live with but can never master. In transactions, in intercourse, whether the gift is of speech or of a harder currency, we seek benchmarks which we will never find. That, too, is a hard truth of—and for—psychoanalysis.

# TRUTH GAMES

## I: Knowing Lies

So I have often reflected on what could have given birth to our scrupulously observed custom of taking bitter offence when we are accused of that vice which is more commonplace among us than any of the others, and why for us it should be the ultimate verbal insult to accuse us of lying. Whereupon I find it natural for us to protect ourselves from those failings with which we are most sullied. It seems that by resenting the accusation and growing angry about it we unload some of the guilt; we are guilty, in fact, but at least we condemn it for show.

Montaigne, "On Giving the Lie"

It is a truism to say that the sciences have developed a privileged claim on truth. The truth of science goes without saying. Other truths—moral, religious, aesthetic, personal—require special pleading, even a special epistemology. Truth, therefore, now has an intimate relation with *knowing* things.

But we should not be too hasty in assuming that the importance attached to truth stems from its recent sequestration by the self-appointed spokespersons of the scientific community. Our devotion to truth is older than the hegemony of science, much to the current benefit of science. For centuries, the concept of truth gained much of its purchase through the conviction that the fate of a man's soul hung on his adherence to the truth. The importance that we in the West attach to truth-telling may well owe much to the importance that the public profession of faith and martyrdom took on in the expanding evangelical origins of the Christian West. Certainly

Augustine's famous preoccupation with lying was in part an attempt to guarantee that one's capacity to bear witness to the truth of Christ not be impaired by any social mores that sanction secret allegiances. The attention to the state of the individual soul required by Christianity demanded an extremely vigilant attitude toward lying. Truth, here, is an ontological and moral question before it is an epistemological one.

Augustine conceived of lying as consisting in a doubling up: saying one thing in speech, and another in one's heart.[1] This doubling conception indicates its affinities with—and reflects its partial origins in—Platonic philosophy, in which the entire dialectic of truth is founded on the doubling, the splitting of appearance and reality. The idea of the truth that lies behind is common both to Platonic conceptions of truth and to the Augustinian conception of lies. But the dialectic of concealing and revealing must stop somewhere, and its end is always on "the other side," the side of reality, rather than appearances. Truth resides "behind" appearances.[2] And the liar conceals the truth in his heart.

When truth becomes hidden behind appearances, the world takes on a depth, becoming a series of layers. Yet the primary and exemplary experience of depth may be that of deception: either that of *being deceived*—by the world or by others—or that of *deceiving* others. The dimension of duplicity, of doubleness, is thus common both to Platonic conceptions of the epistemology of truth, and to moral discussions of the sinfulness of lying. "By means of the lie, consciousness affirms that it exists by nature *as hidden from the Other*,"[3] Sartre observes. Indeed, it may well be lying that gives one the possibility of conceiving of an "appearance" in the first place in the experience of what semblance dissembles. Nor perhaps is it an accident that Augustine's preoccupation with lying was paralleled by his introduction into Christian philosophy of the problem of the existence of "other minds." The original question he posed arose from a consideration of the Last Supper, when Jesus, without naming

8

names, says that one of those around the table will betray him. The problem of other minds arises as the disciples look from one to another, searching out the signs of a betrayal yet to come.[4] And, in the nature of things, each disciple will eventually have to search his own heart, as well as seeking external signs in the demeanor, the appearance of the others.

In this way, the very act of inquiry into the world, the very act of understanding, is seen to involve a duplicity that is akin to that of lying. "The power to deceive is given at the heart of the power to make oneself understood, not as a secondary effect of it, but as its ransom—the other side of the alternative,"[5] writes Jankélévitch. And here a different note is beginning to make itself heard: the note of the creative function of lying. Nietzsche's post-Darwinian argument makes this point more emphatically:

> Insofar as it is a means for the preservation of the individual, the intellect develops its principal forces through dissimulation; the latter is in effect the means through which weaker, less robust individuals survive, given that they are unable to conduct a struggle for existence with horns or the sharp jaw of the beast of prey. In man, this art of dissimulation attains its peak: illusion, flattery, lies and deceit, whispers, posturing, living in borrowed splendor, wearing a mask, hiding behind convention, playing a role for others and oneself . . . are so much the rule and the law among men that there is almost nothing more inconceivable than the arrival of an honest and pure drive for truth among them.[6]

The depth of consciousness created by the exercise of the arts of deception is the first arena for the practice of that dissimulation proper to the life of human intelligence. The same spirit permeates other expositions, for instance that of Karl Popper, who equates the capacity to lie with the capacity to imagine: the power to imagine things other, to *negate*, and thereby to create fiction, even hypothesis—and thence to create science:

The moment when language became human was very closely related to the moment when a man invented a story, a myth in order to excuse a mistake he had made . . . I suggest that the evolution of specifically human language, with its characteristic means of expressing nega- tion—of saying that something signalled is not true—stems very largely from the discovery of systematic means to *negate* false report . . . Indeed it [lying] has made the human language what it is . . . it leads to the *problem of truth or falsity.*[7]

What was an attempt to erect a morality[8] and a theology verges over into a phenomenology—and a naturalistic one at that, in Popper's case—which describes from the inside the development of the capac- ity to lie, and makes of it the mainspring of both human creativity and sin. I will return to explore at greater length this creative function of lying.

This other side of truth may seem a far cry from the assigning of truth functions to formal propositions. But it serves to remind us of the difference between traditional discourses on truth and what has now become the established discourse on scientific truth. Scientific truth does not pay attention to the dilemma or experience of the individual subject—in which deception bulks large. Theories, hy- potheses, and models are taken to exist in their own right, inde- pendent of the subjects who might hold them. Or rather—and this is where the force of the system we call science is said to arise—they are taken to exist solely in relation to what we may call, for simplic- ity's sake, the indivisible, homogeneous, self-identical subject of sci- ence—the subject who is always interchangeable with someone else— the colleague, the peer, *le pair, le semblable, der Mitmensch.*[9] This anonymized, desubjectivized subject can then easily be equated with the social subject, or even the social as subject—when it is argued that the scientific community as an indivisible whole is the knowing subject of science. What is certain is that the transsubjective truth of scientific discourse is evoked whenever one wants to disclaim the implication of the "subjectivity" of any given individual scientific subject in science.

10

On the other hand, in the Western tradition of nonscientific discourse—usually that of ethical and moral discourse—truth is called upon in order to put the subject on the line. This practice runs against the entire metaphysics of Western science. The heritage of the Protestant world of truth with its unique relation to God and His Creation has left indelible marks in the Cartesian grounding, despite the fact that Descartes himself was not Protestant. The brave, defiant "I" despairs of the medieval world constrained entirely within the authority of the Church and Book, yet refuses to join the vociferous skeptics who sweep away every certainty derived from any other source but faith. In its place, it arrives at an equivalent consolatory certainty in the indubitable private world of reason. At the same time, the metaphysics of modern physical science brings Nature as a witness to court. And in the court of natural philosophy, Nature is presumed never to perjure herself—Nature does not deceive.[10]

Descartes secured the certain foundations of modern science by invoking a God who, in his very nature, could not deceive him, Descartes. Descartes thus founds science by placing this crucial constraint upon the nature of God. Einstein founds his science—restricting the sort of physics he would regard as acceptable—by placing an analogous restraint upon God's nature: "Subtle is the Lord, but malicious he is not."[11] For Descartes, observing the constitutional inadequacy of man's sensory and intellectual equipment, the skeptical challenge came to a head in the possibility of *being deceived*. The active deception of Descartes's malicious demon is simply a focus for the more general and chronic threat of being deceived, despite one's efforts to make the best of one's equipment. The demon's counterpart, the non-deceiving God, allows at least one or two certainties to be laid down across the swamp of potential self-deception. The crucial step here is the elimination of *malicious* deception.

The project of escaping from the human world of appearances and deception, even from the pettiness of passion and strife, did not always express itself, as it did for Descartes, in an epistemology that defeated the threat of deception. With the development of science

11

as an institution and a social ideal, the desire to escape from the human into truth could be viewed simply as a deep, personal motive. As Einstein wrote:

> I believe with Schopenhauer that one of the strongest motives that lead persons to art and science is flight from everyday life, with its painful harshness and wretched dreariness, and from the fetters of one's own shifting desires . . . With this negative motive there goes a positive one. Man seeks to form for himself, in whatever manner is suitable for him, a simplified and lucid image of the world, and so to overcome the world of experience by striving to replace it to some extent by this image.[12]

But in the sixteenth and seventeenth centuries, the urgency of finding some grounds for certainty clearly did not stem from the need to find a proto-ideology for a science that did not as yet exist, but rather from the requirements of religion and morals. These discourses about truth may not originally have been primarily concerned with knowledge so much as with ethical questions. And as old as the debates about skepticism are the tirades launched against lying, the practice that undermines the possibility of truth from within. An examination of these tirades will help us to see more clearly the issues underlying the discourses on truth, whether they are "epistemological" or "ethical."

---

> For fifteen years I was the world's best faker. Honestly—they should have a phallic trophy—mounted on a pedestal (like in the art history books) for *all women*—I think they all fake it with men.
>
> *The Hite Report*

Extremism of conclusion and extremism of argument have been the characteristics of philosophical views of lying.[13] Augustine regarded lying as a mortal sin, since the doubleness of deceitful speech—having one thing in one's heart, saying another—subverted the God-given purpose of speech: to tell the truth.[14] This Augustinian concentration on the intention to deceive held sway in Aquinas's reiteration and reformulation pretty much until the seventeenth century. It is worth considering the context of Augustine's hard line.

His major discussions of lying occur in *De mendacio* (On Lying) of 395 and *Contra mendacium* (Against Lying) of 420. The first enunciated the doctrine of the intention to deceive;[15] but the second text, when placed in its context, is far more revealing of the issues at stake in lying. The occasion for the writing of this tract was the emergence of the Priscillianist heresy, which included the doctrine that lying is sometimes justified, especially in order to conceal religious doctrines from strangers. Augustine was quick to point out that a consequence of this doctrine would be that one would not be able to tell who was a Priscillianist and who wasn't. Indeed, certain zealous Catholics pretended to be Priscillianists in order to discover who the Priscillianists were, including one, Consentius, who asked Augustine to comment on this "pious fraud" as a means of detecting the heretics.

The Priscillianists argued that speaking the truth in one's heart was sufficient—there was no necessity for speaking it out loud.[16] As so often, Augustine's arguments advising Consentius center upon the egotistical task of saving one's own soul; the Priscillianist doctrines are mistakes, not lies. Hence: "For, what they say when they are lying is one thing; what they say when they are mistaken is another. When they teach their heresy, they say those things about which they are mistaken."[17] In consequence, if one believes their professed dogmas, one dies (that is, one goes to Hell), whereas if one believes them to be Catholics when in fact they are not, one does not put one's own soul at risk.[18] Following their doctrine on lying will ensure that true Catholicism is no longer visible. But if Catholics profess their, the Priscillianists', dogmas in order to catch them, those who hear may end in death. That is, once one permits that first lie, for whatever purpose, the outcome becomes *uncertain*—when you reveal yourselves to them, they will not know what to believe, since they know that you are a liar.

Augustine's attack on this doctrine[19] indicates how truth for him was conceived of as identical with the eternal nature of God: God and truth are the same thing. The notion that truth supplies a stable reference point, taking over this function in philosophical discourse from the function that God has in theological discourse, is a crucial theme in the historical dialectic of lying and truth. The other great hard-liner in the history of lying, Immanuel Kant, clearly testifies to this.

The background to Kant's argument is to be found in Grotius's reformulation of doctrines of truthfulness in terms of natural law, endorsed by Benjamin Constant, whom Kant was criticizing. It is only wrong to lie to those who have a right to the truth, Constant argued. To lie to those who do not belong to the society is not a transgression of the social contract. But the argument produces a slippage: what the contract thus amounts to, and what society now amounts to, is a convention, a *rule* (rather than a natural law) of truthfulness, whose only guarantee is the social itself. Society now takes the place of God as guarantor of truth. And, as we shall see, the Priscillianist heresy can emerge in a new and different form.

The core of Kant's reply was this: no lies are admissible, since in lying one denies one's own humanity, that is, one denies one's right to one's own truthfulness.[20] It is not a question of whether or not one harms the other to whom one lies: "For a lie always harms another; if not some other particular man, still it harms mankind generally, for it vitiates the source of law itself . . . truthfulness is a duty which must be regarded as the ground of all duties based on contract, and the laws of these duties would be rendered uncertain and useless if even the least exception to them were admitted."[21] This passion against the possible subversion of contractual obligation is reminiscent of the practice of Quakers, who banned all speech during the agreement of contracts in order to make clear the relation of the speaker to his peers and to God the Witness.

Kant's arguments are somewhat surprising, not only for their unbending condemnation of all falsehood, but for their displacement of the raison d'être of the argument onto other indispensable institutions: the law and contractual obligation. Each statement that one makes is akin to the proverbial finger in the dike—let one lie pass, and the whole of the commonwealth will be flooded. But the ultimate reason for not removing one's finger from the dike is evidently a pragmatic one. Indeed, many arguments demonstrating the evils of lying take the form of a deduction: imagine a society in which such acts were permitted—then you will immediately see that such a society can no longer function. Perhaps Kant also had in mind as his target that form of enlightened paternalistic elitism associated with an earlier generation of *philosophes,* epitomized in Voltaire's request to his philosophical allies: "A lie is a vice only when it does harm," he wrote in 1736, "it is a very great virtue when it does good. So, be more virtuous than ever. You must lie like a devil, not timidly, not for a while, but boldly, and persistently . . . Lie, my friends, lie, I shall repay you when I get the chance."[22]

While Kant's argument may have a certain force—enjoining as much or as little assent as we would give to the assertion that our society could not function without electrical engineers—it is not very deep. Some of the work of criticizing the conflation of the moral condemnation of lying with a description of the prerequisites for smooth social functioning had already been accomplished by David Hume, with his habitual penetration and skepticism. In his treatise *The Religion of Nature Delineated* (1722), William Wollaston had argued that all wrongdoing is a species of lying—the representation of what is false. Thus stealing is misrepresenting what belongs to someone else as belonging to oneself; adultery is misrepresenting someone else's wife as one's own. Hume replied to Wollaston that, according to such an argument, adultery committed in secret, not giving rise to a misrepresentation (to others), would not be wrong. And this leads to the heart of the matter: conceiving all immorality as a subspecies of lying, denying how things are, leaves unanswered the major question: why is falsehood wrong? This is the famous unbridgeable gulf—between *is* and *ought,* between a society with or without electrical engineers, with or without truthsayers. Without a

15

moral grounding for the condemnation of lying, the moralist is left with a functionalist argument: society could not function if everyone told lies. And this position—"What if everybody told lies?"—invites Groucho Marx's riposte: "Then I'd be a fool not to!"

———

> The former are convinced that among the false books flooding the world they can track down the few that bear a truth perhaps extra-human or extra-terrestrial. The latter believe that only counterfeiting, mystification, intentional falsehood can represent absolute value in a book, a truth not contaminated by the dominant pseudo truths.
>
> Italo Calvino, *If on a Winter's Night a Traveler*

The very idea of a society based on lying is repeatedly asserted to be self-contradictory. Sir Thomas Browne declared that "so large is the Empire of Truth, that it hath place within the wall of Hell, and the Devils themselves are daily forced to practice it; . . . although they deceive us, they lie not unto each other; as well understanding that all community is continued by Truth, and that of Hell cannot consist without it."[23] Rather than assuming that truth is the foundation of any possible commerce between people, what would it be like to countenance—in an equable manner, rather than donning the cloak of the *enfant terrible*—the symmetry of truth and lies, and the possibility of a society based on lies rather than truth? Could such a methodological principle, derived from the working practices of anthropologists, imported into the history and philosophy of science by Bloor[24] and others, be countenanced, let alone found effective?

Alexandre Koyré did not take it as axiomatic that society could not be based on a lie. In "Réflexions sur le mensonge," published in 1942 when he was in exile in New York, he attempted to analyze such a society—reflections bearing, one surmises, like the other two powerful contemporary treatises on lying by Sartre and Jankélévitch, directly upon the state of truth to be found in Vichy France. Koyré's analysis starts with an anthropological claim: "It is certain that man is defined by speech, that the latter brings with it the possibility of lying and that—pace Porphyry—the lie, much more than the laugh, is what is unique to man."[25] Lying, he continues, like the laugh, is the favored weapon of the oppressed—to fool the oppressor is to humiliate him. Under what conditions will lying become acceptable? Koyré asks.

His answer is given in terms of the relation of the subject and the other, of "us" and "them." Societies that tolerate lying are those in which conflict and heterogeneity are paramount; persecution from "outside" is necessary for the lie to become a fundamental part of the order of society. In particular, it presupposes contact between hostile elements of different societies—a mythical, agonistically social state of nature, prior to the constitution of "true" society. In order to cohere, this ideal society requires a firm base, which we might as well call the truth. But, in the face of a hostile world, the lie will have to become the principle of the existence of the society. As a consequence, the society will, in the limiting case, now disappear in the eyes of the others. The society disappears into the night of the secret. "Hence, a total inversion has taken place: the lie, become the group secret, will be the condition of its existence, its habitual mode of being, fundamental and primary."[26] The perfect Priscillianist society has now come into existence. To quote Koyré again:

> As a consequence, the supreme duty of a member of this secret grouping, the act in which he expresses his attachment and his faithfulness to the group, the act by which he affirms and confirms his adhesion to the group, consists, paradoxically, in his dissimulation of this fact. To dissimulate what is and in order to be able to do so, simulate what isn't: such is the mode of existence that, necessarily, all secret societies impose upon their members.[27]

Once constituted, then, a social grouping will, given a hostile environment, necessarily constitute itself anew not as a secret society, but as something more profound—what Koyré calls "une société à secret," a society *of* the secret, a society whose existence is now predicated upon the secret. And complete loss of foundations seems to follow from here. Does it exist? How could one possibly detect its existence? From what standpoint could one determine the existence of both an inside and an outside to such a society?

Koyré indicates how such a society would bring into existence an entirely new topography of the relations of the lie and the truth. No member of such a society will believe what the leader says, knowing that public pronouncements are for the benefit of the others. But, equally, it is possible for the leader to make use of this rhetorical move to employ the double lie: saying the truth because he knows it will not be believed by the "others," and only in a manner of speaking by "us"—the classic example is *Mein Kampf*. But even in the 1920s, American social psychological studies implied that there already existed delinquent sub-societies of this character, "a social order whose very foundation is its negation."[28] Certainly those bureaucracies whose ethos is the Weberian ethic of responsibility are likely to produce a high official who can jestingly ask: "What is truth?" and not wait for an answer.

Thus far I have treated the problem of lying as being a matter of all or nothing. That is not the most common way to approach it, since there is something privatizing and individualizing in lying that prompts us to think more in terms of "some lying" than "everything is lies" or "nobody should lie." Hume indicated, with his habitual teasing wit, how Kant's argument in the form he offered it, that lying vitiates the source of law and the stability of contractual obligation, fares rather poorly in this light:

> And though it is allowed that, without a regard to property, no society could subsist; yet according to the imperfect way in which human affairs are conducted, a sensible knave, in particular incidents, may think that an act of iniquity or infidelity will make a considerable addition to his fortune, without causing a considerable breach in the social union and confederacy. That *honest is the best policy*, may be a good general rule, but is liable to many exceptions; and he, it may perhaps be thought, conducts himself with most wisdom, who observes the general rule, and takes advantage of all the exceptions.[29]

18

It is not the law-abiding citizen that is the problem, but the "sensible knave," the "free rider," the subject of rational decision theory, or the "bad man" of Oliver Wendell Holmes's positivist essay on the path of the law.[30] One hears behind the zealousness of Kant's condemnation of lying the hushed departure of God from the debate over lying, already signaled by Montaigne's acute observation (in the splendid version of Francis Bacon): "If it be well weighed, to say that a man lieth, is as much to say, as that he is brave towards God and a coward towards men." If there is no God, the liar is not obliged to be brave toward anyone.

The critique of the absolutist position on lying focuses first on the givens of human life: it proposes an anthropology of lying, opposing the absolutist condemnation with an account of lying's universal human function. We have already encountered the first defense of lying: the notion that the dissimulation and deceit of the liar are an expression of virtue. These are the virtues embodied for the Greeks in Odysseus: cunning, craftiness, and astuteness.

> What did the Greeks admire in Odysseus? Above all, his capacity for lying, and for cunning and terrible retribution; his being equal to contingencies; when need be, appearing nobler than the noblest; the ability to be *whatever he chose;* heroic perseverance; having all means at his command; possession of intellect—his intellect is the admiration of the gods, they smile when they think of it—: all this is the Greek *ideal!* The most remarkable thing about it is that the antithesis of appearance and being is not felt at all and is thus of no significance morally. Have there ever been such consummate actors![31]

Here the lie is a maneuver carried out in order to retain control of a situation, managing the play of appearances, of doubleness for strategic ends.[32] Touchstone, one of Shakespeare's theorists of the gradation of lies, "uses his folly like a stalking-horse, and under the presentation of that he shoots his wit."[33] So lying comes to appear not as a perversion of language, but as its perfection for pragmatic ends. As a contemporary linguist puts it: "It might even be claimed that the ultimate goal of language acquisition is to lie effectively . . . real lying . . . is the deliberate use of language as a tool . . . to mislead the listener."[34] Evolutionary biologists debate the selectionist advantages of truth-telling over lying—arguing, for instance, that an animal that, programmed by a deceiving gene, deceived others by not giving warning calls would eventually take over the group, but that this group would then be at a disadvantage relative to other groups characterized by truth-telling, altruistic behavior.[35]

It is the liars who know best how most of us conduct ourselves in relation to truth. Nietzsche observes: "One says what one thinks, one is 'truthful' only under certain conditions: namely, that one is understood (*inter pares*), and understood with good will (once again *inter pares*). One conceals oneself in presence of the unfamiliar: and he who wants to attain something says what he would like to have thought of him, but *not* what he thinks. ('The powerful always lie.')"[36] Truth-telling is reserved for relations of equality or even for relations of intimacy and equality—an instructive juxtaposition with the political and economic theory of sovereign, equal, self-determining subjects, the theory of bourgeois individualism. Out there, in society, in the name of both one's own interests and those of society, one dissembles. "I've always recognized that if one spoke one's mind for just one minute, society would crumble," noted Sainte-Beuve.[37] The variations on dissembling indicate the complexities of social relations: to one's equals, one employs irony, the mask that is intended to be unmasked, like a secret code, whereas for one's inferiors and superiors one presents the blank screen of the lie.[38] If lying is thought to make society impossible, it is irony that facilitates understanding in social circumstances of considerable friction and conflict. And then there are etiquette, white lies, and lovers' lies—these are the oil that keeps the motor of our relations with others from seizing up:

> When my love swears she is made of truth,
> I do believe her though I know she lies.

20

That she might think me some untutored youth,
Unlearnèd in the world's false subtleties.

. . . . .

Therefore I lie with her, and she with me,
And in our faults by lies we flattered be.[39]

Then there are the necessities of exaggeration—distortions and exaggerations that are required to communicate the truth:

That staircase . . . seemed to me a thing so marvellous that I told my parents that it was an antique staircase brought from ever so far away by M. Swann. My regard for the truth was so great that I should not have hesitated to give them this information even if I had known it to be false, for it alone could enable them to feel for the dignity of the Swanns' staircase the same respect that I felt myself—just as when one is talking to some ignorant person who cannot understand what constitutes the genius of a great doctor, it is well not to admit that he does not know how to cure a cold in the head.[40]

Those who acknowledge that the requirements of "truth" demand that one lie in her service betray their impatience with the sentimental, with the idealist and the naive who call for sincerity from their intimates:

I hate questioners and questions; there are so few that can be spoken to without a lie. *'Do you forgive me?'* Madam and sweetheart, so far as I have gone in life I have never yet been able to discover what forgiveness means. *'Is it still the same between us?'* Why, how can it be? It is eternally different; and yet you are still the friend of my heart. *'Do you understand me?'* God knows; I should think it highly improbable.[41]

The ease with which we lie can even be breathtakingly disarming in the display of its uncomplicated social virtue: "Yes, I always fake orgasms. It just seems polite. Why be rude?"[42]

The fundamental paternalism (or is it maternalism?) of the liar—

most evident, ironically enough, in the woman who fakes orgasm in the best interests of all concerned—raises a new question: could it ever be, indeed could it always be, in my best interests to be deceived rather than told the truth? Utilitarian theory certainly countenances such a possibility. Hume asserted that "morals must always be handled with a view to public interest, more than philosophical regularity."[43] Bentham makes explicit that the considerations of public interest deprive the question of truth and lying of any moral dimension beyond that of harm to others: "Falsehood, take it by itself, consider it as not being accompanied by any other material circumstances, nor therefore productive of any material effects, can never, upon the principle of utility, constitute any offence at all."[44] The utilitarian arguments were directed primarily at the public spheres of law and government, but their form can, as Proust noted, be completely generalized: "So much did she enjoy giving pleasure that she had come to employ a particular kind of falsehood peculiar to certain utilitarians and men who have 'arrived.' Existing, incidentally, in an embryonic state in a vast number of people, this form of insincerity consists in not being able to confine the pleasure arising out of a single act of politeness to a single person."[45] The division of labor may be between ruler and ruled or between lover and beloved. Jonathan Swift dryly portrayed the fundamental contrasting positions as being those of the knave and the fool; given the choice, it was, he made clear, certainly preferable to be the fool:

> In the proportion that credulity is a more peaceful possession of the mind than curiosity, so far preferable is that wisdom that converses about the surface to that pretended philosophy which enters into the depth of things, and then comes gravely back with informations and discoveries that in the inside they are good for nothing . . . And he whose fortunes and dispositions have placed him in a convenient station to . . . content his ideas with films and images that fly off upon his senses from the superfices of things; such a man, truly wise, creams off nature, leaving the sour and the dregs for philosophy and reason to lap up. This is the sublime and refined point of felicity, called the

22

possession of being well deceived; the serene peaceful state of being a fool among knaves.[46]

Are peace and contentment a higher good than truthfulness, sincerity, and openness? Or, more forcefully, is truthfulness irredeemably compromised by its association with blindness, callous cruelty, and the pointless pursuit of knowledge for its own sake?

Beyond the question of the competing virtues and their relation to lying is the claim that lying is creative—as in Proust's reflection:

> The lie, the perfect lie, about people we know, about the relations we have had with them, about our motive for some action, formulated in totally different terms, the lie as to what we are, whom we love, what we feel with regard to people who love us and believe that they have fashioned us in their own image because they keep on kissing us morning, noon and night—that lie is one of the few things in the world that can open windows for us on to what is new and unknown, that can awaken in us sleeping senses for the contemplation of universes that otherwise we should never have known.[47]

Such lying awakens us to the unknown, the mystery of the other. We live most easily in a state of somnolence, a complacent inattention, from which the falsehoods of our intimates awaken us. In the dialectic between the real and the possible, lying plays an indispensable role. "Words ought to be a little wild—for they are the assault of thoughts upon the unthinking," wrote Keynes.[48] An indubitable sign of autism in a child, it is claimed by psychologists, is the inability to hide, to dissemble, to deceive or to lie.[49] Without these capacities, the possibility of other minds is foreclosed. "Faced with the structural rigor of the real, he loses all notion of the possible"[50]—this is the philosopher's description of an aphasic who could speak but not lie.

The lies of childhood have a peculiar mystery and fascination; they have certainly been a major preoccupation of spiritual guides and those psychologists who took on the mantle of the priests. The unintended consequences of such spiritual concern are also wryly

23

educational—"I was brought up in a clergyman's household so I am a first-class liar," confessed Sybil Thorndike. Another theatrical child of a professionally religious home, Ingmar Bergman, traced his compulsive story-telling, his art, to this fact:

> Nowadays, I understand my parents' desperation. A pastor's family lives as if on a tray, unprotected from other eyes. The parsonage must always be open to criticism and comments from the congregation. Both Father and Mother were perfectionists who sagged beneath this unreasonable pressure . . . I think I came off [better than my siblings] by turning myself into a liar. I created an external person who had very little to do with the real me. As I didn't know how to keep my creation and my person apart, the damage had consequences for my life and creativity far into adulthood. Sometimes I have to console myself with the fact that he who has lived a lie loves the truth.[51]

Lying is always distinguished from error or falsity by its deliberateness. When we consider the lies of children, or when we remember our childhood lies, it is the characteristic of willed autonomy that often strikes us. As Jankélévitch puts it, "if sin, far from being error, is something one commits on purpose, the lie becomes the sin *par excellence,* not necessarily the most serious, but the most characteristic, the quintessence of sin. Because one never lies without willing it. Hence the gravity of the first lie of an infant. The day of this first lie is a truly solemn day where we discover in the innocent the disturbing depth of *'conscience.'*"[52] The memory of one's childhood lies persists and may take on mythical or allegorical dimensions. As so often when children are discussed, researchers are engaged in the search for origins, finding in the first lie the first glimmerings of consciousness, independence, sin, or even a self.

The search for origins notoriously haunted the encounter of Europeans with their others, the natives of other lands. In European travelers' tales and stories of far-off lands, the mirroring and projection processes are enmeshed with seeking the origins of civilization, morality, and nobility in the split between self and other. Lying, whose inherent structure reveals the duplicity of consciousness, lends itself particularly well to the seesaw dynamics of all such mirroring encounters with the other, the native, as we find them explored and deconstructed in Montaigne's famous essay on cannibals, where he noted: "Among them you hear no words for treachery, lying, cheating, avarice, envy, backbiting or forgiveness . . . no opinion has ever been so unruly as to justify treachery, disloyalty, tyranny and cruelty, which are everyday vices in us. So we can indeed call those folk barbarians by the rules of reason but not in comparison with ourselves, who surpass them in every kind of barbarism."[53] One hundred years later, in 1686, Ten Rhyne wrote in his journal of his encounter with the Hottentots: "In faithlessness, inconstancy, lying, cheating, treachery, and infamous concern with every kind of lust they [the Hottentots] exercise their villainy." Meeting the same people a few years later, Grevenbrock reflected: "From us they have learned blasphemy, perjury, strife, quarrelling, drunkenness, trickery . . . misdeeds unknown to them before, and among other crimes of deepest die, the accursed lust for gold."[54]

The dialectic between traveler and native is repeated in our stories of childhood innocence and experience. An old lady told me the following story. "I remember when I was a little girl, my mother told me that she could always tell when people were lying by looking into their eyes. I lived in fear of this awesome power of my mother's, until one day, on coming home from school—I must have been five or six—I was chatting with my mother, when some delicate topic came up and, with great fear and trepidation, I told her a lie. My mother seemed to look into my eyes and then turn away, apparently not noticing anything. From that moment on, a great burden was taken from my shoulders." This lie was her first act of independence. We might say that the lie revealed to the little girl that she herself truly had a mind that was other to her mother's. The depth of her own consciousness revealed itself in her mother's lack of awareness.

This creative function of the lie, linked with the possibility of otherness, the very possibility of possibility, appears to be a natural function, one whose absence is viewed as pathology. In early twentieth century literature on lying in children, written primarily from an educational and moralistic standpoint, the question is asked whether children under a given age can lie, shifting from the age of four[55] to as young as fifteen months in the more recent literature.[56] But, significantly, lying is often redescribed as something else: "In the first five years, children do not speak truths or falsehoods, all they do is speak."[57] And then, as if regretting the loss of the moral condemnation of lying that such naturalism entails, the "natural" posture of moral opprobrium may be reinstated.

There is a conflict here between different languages of description—between an epistemological claim and a moral ascription. The epistemological claim is that the lie of the child is an index of the possibility of thinking *against* the real, of counterfactuality, of hypothesis, of the imaginary. The fact that it is perceived, described, and conceived of as a lie indicates that the first field of epistemological activity is the social field—knowledge is initially intimately bound up with our relations to others. At the same time, there are the moral discourses which, as we have seen, regard lying with, at the very least, circumspection. The field of lying is thus always under tension.

Yet there is a distinctive institution in Western society which occupies this contested field: the institution of fiction. Itself an answer to the problems of elaborating moral discourses in the early modern period, fiction gives up its claim to represent the real, while at the same time it leaves hanging in delicious suspense the question of what exactly its representative function is. As Hume noted, "poets . . . though liars by profession, always endeavor to give an air of truth to their fictions,"[58] so it should come as no surprise that fiction is a privileged site for the inquiry into the epistemology, morality, and pragmatics of lying. As should already be evident, it is writers of fiction who demonstrate the delicacies, complexities, and ironies of lying most clearly—and it is writers like Proust who can best do justice to La Rochefoucauld's observation that "truth does less good in the world than its appearances do harm." The ability of Proust's masterpiece to swerve away from reality and then shadow it so convincingly, beginning with the indeterminate relation of the narrator to the author, demonstrates how fiction achieves its aim of pinning down the real while never claiming reality for itself. The Ionian word for truth means "openly," and that for lie means "curved."[59] Fiction takes the curved path, the swerve of the lie, telling it "slant" so as to arrive at "The Truth's superb surprise."[60]

When one attempts to assess the world-historical function of fiction, the most plausible answers come in mythical form. Freud told a story—myth thinly disguised—in which the poet was the first liar and thus the first man who had the courage to be an individual. After the murder of the primal father, Freud recounted, the constitutional premise of the society thus created was that no man put himself in the place of the dead father. Instead, each male placed the dead father in the position of his ideal. The first man to free himself from this requirement of submission to the dead father did so out of his longing for and his desire to be the father, through a feat of his imagination:

> This poet disguised the truth with lies in accordance with his longing. He invented the heroic myth. The hero was a man who by himself had slain the father—the father who still appeared in the myth as a totemic monster . . . The myth, then, is the step by which the individual emerges from group psychology. The first myth was certainly the psychological, the hero myth; the explanatory nature myth must have followed much later. The poet who had taken this step and had in this way set himself free from the group in his imagination, is nevertheless able . . . to find his way back to it in reality. For he goes and relates to the group his hero's deeds which he has invented. At bottom this hero is no one but himself. Thus he lowers himself to the level of reality, and raises his hearers to the level of imagination. But his hearers understand the poet, and, in virtue of their having the same relation of longing towards the primal father, they can identify themselves with the hero.[61]

Freud's account makes the "first" individual double: on the one hand, he is the hero, who is above the complexity of lying, an Achilles who "hates him like the gates of death who thinks one thing and says another" and who therefore "speaks that which shall be accomplished,"[62] the hero who is often portrayed (like Siegfried in Wagner's *Ring*, who has never passed from the megalomania of infancy to the human state of fearfulness) as too innocent, too animal-like in his natural gifts, to be capable of deception.[63] And at the same time, shadowing the hero, there is the poet, whose individuality emerges in the lie he tells. If Plato's account counterposes Achilles the truthsayer and Odysseus the liar, Freud's account discloses that Achilles is Homer's cover and stand-in, so that the true hero, Achilles, is seen as nothing but a ploy of the poet's. It is the liar, the poet, who conceals himself under the cover of the myth of the hero. The hero is the poet in disguise. Certainly, the hero is doubled by his creator, who masquerades as his mere servant, a messenger. And we have to see Achilles as the more worked character than the true-to-life Odysseus, Homer's companion in wily fictionality, because the honest and straightforward truthsayer stands that much further away from the truth. In this doubling function of the poet, we come upon the inherent structure of truth and appearance, now pinpointed in Freud's myth as the origin of the individual.

---

> Overheard through open window on U.S. college campus: "Suck, I said, suck it!—blow is only an expression!"
>
> Losey Latin

What fiction and these founding myths achieve is a systematic confusion of lies and truth. One of the boldest accounts of the foundational intermingling of truth and lies, that in Nietzsche's early essay "On Truth and Lies in the Extramoral Sense," achieves this end by grounding truth on lies—not out of a quixotic attempt to *épater la vérité*, as it might be fair to describe Oscar Wilde's splendid essay *The Decay of Lying*, but out of Nietzsche's quest for a higher, more credible seat of judgment than truth. The project is summed up well in a passage from *The Will to Power*: "If the morality of 'thou shalt not lie' is rejected, the 'sense for truth' will have to legitimize itself before another tribunal:—as a means of the preservation of man, as *will to power.*"[64]

Nietzsche's naturalistic myth opens with the presocial individual using his intellect for dissimulation in his incessant skirmishes with other individuals. But, "from boredom and necessity," he seeks peace; the peace treaty he enters into brings with it a *convention:* "a uniformly valid and binding designation is invented for things, and this legislation of language likewise establishes the first laws of truth."[65] The unpleasant consequences of lying—characterized, with shades of Wollaston, as "using the valid designations, the words, in order to make something which is unreal appear to be real"—are now excluded, and "man now wants nothing but truth: he desires the pleasant, life-preserving consequences of truth."[66] Nietzsche has thus explained one fundamental fact: the human drive for truth.

Nietzsche is quick to dispel the notion that this convention and this drive for truth are anything like what philosophers understand as truth—an adequate representation of the real. "The various languages placed side by side show that with words it is never a question of truth, never a question of adequate expression; otherwise, there would not be so many languages."[67] From the sheer diversity, resilience, and efficiency of the thousands of languages people use, it is clear that language has very little to do with truth. In a Wittgensteinian moment, we might say that all of these languages are just so many truth games.

So what is truth? . . . truths are illusions we have forgotten are illusions; they are metaphors which have become habitual and drained of sensory force, coins which have been effaced and which from then on are taken to be, not pieces of money, but metal . . . so far we have heard only of the duty which society imposes in order to exist: to be truthful means to employ the usual metaphors. Thus, to express it morally, this is the duty to lie according to a fixed convention, to lie with the herd and in a manner binding upon everyone. To be sure, man forgets that things are like this for him; so he lies unconsciously in the required manner and in accordance with age-old custom—and, precisely because of this unconsciousness and this forgetting, he arrives at a feeling of truth.[68]

Given this Hobbesian vision of society, the lie becomes an instrument of that highest good—peace and understanding between men. Truth is thus the convention, the lie, by which we live with one another in peace.

There is another naturalistic argument, having some affinities with Nietzsche's, that recognizes that truth-telling needs no defense; it therefore does not need to follow Augustine, Kant, and the moralists in exiling the liar as the ultimate danger to society. However, instead of telling a story of the elaboration of truth games out of lies and compromise, this argument simply identifies a natural truth-telling disposition in mankind, a disposition which, being natural, is to be neither praised nor condemned. The obverse of this naturalistic coin is the recognition of the equally natural disposition to lie. Thus, if it is natural for humans to seek truth, any critique of lying would be misplaced, since what is natural needs no defense. There are, in particular, no *a priori* arguments concerning the virtue of truth.

Hume puts this argument well: "Were not the memory tenacious to a certain degree; had not men commonly an inclination to truth and a principle of probity; were they not sensible to shame, when detected in a falsehood: Were not these, I say, discovered by *experience* to be qualities, inherent in human nature, we should never repose the least confidence in human testimony."[69] We can extend Hume's relaxed observation of the dominant but by no means universal tendency to tell the truth. If truth-telling needs no underpinning, then the institutions of promising and of contractual obligation need no underpinning. The predominant practice of Anglo-American courts, perhaps taking their historical cue from the cynical wisdom of the Scottish Enlightenment, would seem to bear this out:

True, fraud, misrepresentation and duress must be ruled out by the courts in the exercise of their function of making sure that the "rules of the game" will be adhered to. But these categories were narrowly defined (at least by the nineteenth century common law) due to the strong belief in the policing force of the market. Oppressive bargains, it was taken for granted, can be avoided by careful shopping around. Contracting parties are expected to look out for their own interest and their own protection. "Let the bargainer beware," as we were told, was (and to some extent still is) the ordinary rule of contract. It is not the function of courts to strike down improvident bargains. Courts have only to interpret contracts made by the parties. They do not make them.[70]

This relaxed, laissez-faire attitude to truth-telling and deception may not altogether satisfy us. If truth-telling is seen as a "natural disposition" it becomes tempting to compare it to another natural disposition, sexuality, which is also an assemblage of activities that are massively policed and contested. In this light, would truth-telling be like heterosexuality, and would lying, deception, and dissimulation be like homosexuality, sadism, and all the other perversions?

If so, restoring to these "perversions" their rights as natural acts or the result of natural dispositions is not likely to leave things as they are; one would be tempted to interrogate each of these different natural dispositions, including the dominant natural disposition, along the lines of the question that Freud puts to conventional heterosexuality: "the exclusive sexual interest felt by men for women is also a problem that needs elucidating and is not a self-evident fact based upon an attraction that is ultimately of a chemical nature."[71] The parallel would inevitably lead to viewing truth-telling—and, in particular, compulsive and "exclusive" truth-telling—as a problem that needs elucidating. Nietzsche's more astringent genealogical naturalism is in part devoted to that problem. Despite arguments that find an asymmetry between truth and lying in the observation that telling the truth never raises questions about one's motives, whereas telling lies always does,[72] there is every reason to be curious about truth-telling and its manifold guises and institutions. For a start, one can love truth out of the murkiest of motives, as Proust, also taking his analogy from the field of sexual behavior, points out: "No doubt, as [Swann] used to assure Odette, he loved sincerity, but only as he might love a pimp who could keep him in touch with the daily life of his mistress."[73]

The fully developed Kantian ethics founded upon the concept of the categorical imperative demands that each person be treated as an end and not as a means.[74] Alasdair MacIntyre interprets this as overlapping the distinction between manipulative and nonmanipulative social relations.[75] It is wrong to tell a lie because that treats the other as a means, not an end. But it does not take much experience of the world to recognize that telling the truth can be equally manipulative. To take one contemporary example, consider the use of statistics and medical "findings," as they are euphemistically called, for whipping up health scares, now a perennial part of the biopolitical truth games of Western societies. Such media-saturating "truth scares," as we might call them, are as much in the service of interested parties in the medical-industrial complex (including those politicians and "responsible authorities" attempting to cover their backs, in accordance with an intricate actuarial calculation, against every possible future—and past—eventuality) as they are designed to promote the health of the population at large—itself a complex and contested category. So it would be more faithful to social reality to invoke Marx's portrait of the free bourgeois subjects who, in contractual relations, *necessarily* treat each other as means, not ends, and then, as if their reading of Kant had given them a bad conscience, later console themselves with the symmetry of the relation. I treat someone as a means, but he treats me similarly, so that the common interest "proceeds, as it were, behind the back of these self-reflected particular interests, behind the back of one individual's interest in opposition to that of the other."[76]

Hence, far from it always being "natural" to credit the other with the lack of motive, the disinterestedness, with which truth-telling requires itself to be associated, it is only by employing a rhetorical technique that the speaker can begin to lay claim to the truth-effect.

This rhetorical technique consists in turning the attention of the hearer away from the motivational or social context of the utterance. As Elster reflects: "In the hands of the apologist, good reasons are transformed into tools of persuasion. The recipient is in a bind, for should he listen to the reasons or to the tone of voice in which they are advanced? It takes more than ordinary good faith to be susceptible to good reasons advanced in bad faith."[77]

It may, at this point, be consolatory to reflect that games in which the truth counts—and hence ones in which lying is possible, ones which are signposted for us as lying games—are limited, albeit special ones. And, in this world, subject to change and chance, today's truth-teller may be tomorrow's liar, and vice versa. As Charlie Noble, a character in Hermann Melville's *The Confidence-Man,* remarks: "There is no bent of heart or turn of thought which any man holds by virtue of an unalterable nature or will. Even those feelings and opinions deemed most identical with eternal right and truth, it is not impossible but that, as personal persuasions, they may in reality be but the result of some chance tip of Fate's elbow in throwing her dice."[78]

If truth-telling ends up as a chance tip of Fate's elbow, then trust too needs to be considered as a similar disposition, perhaps even an instinctual disposition. If trust is instinctual, it renders implausible the idea that one could *choose* to trust the other. Perhaps truth-telling and truth-hearing are akin to those states of mind that Elster has pinpointed as being inherently unavailable as objects of choice. One cannot, in his exemplary case, choose to be spontaneous. Can one choose to trust another person? Those acts that appear exemplary of trust, such as lending money or promising to love and to cherish, are enactments of trust rather than being founded on a decision to trust (or not, as the case may be).

As J. L. Austin pointed out in *How to Do Things with Words,* it is misleading to interpret such utterances as "I promise" as derivative of inner mental states of promising or trusting. There is nothing *beyond* such utterances that makes them trustworthy. Trust and confidence may easily be attributes like balance or grace that disappear once they are put in question and examined for their foundations. Confidence may well be just a confidence-trick—another form of Nietzsche's seemingly paradoxical account of truth as based on lying. This would not prevent trust and confidence from being allied with, being shored up by, being braced by, being inextricably fated to stand or fall with other institutions.[79] One obvious candidate institution in this family is money. As Marx noted in his acerbic way:

> The existence of money presupposes the objectification [*Versachlichung*] of the social bond; in so far, that is, as money appears in the form of *collateral* which one individual must leave with another in order to obtain a commodity from him. Here the economists themselves say that people place in a thing (money) the faith which they do not place in each other. But why do they have faith in the thing? Obviously only because that thing is an *objectified relation* between persons; because it is objectified exchange value, and exchange value is nothing more than a mutual relation between people's productive activities. Every other collateral may serve the holder directly in that function: money serves him only as the "dead pledge of society,"[80] but it serves as such only because of its social (symbolic) property; and it can have a social property only because individuals have alienated their own social relationship from themselves so that it takes the form of a thing.[81]

Money becomes a guarantee because there is conscious bad faith, distrust, and suspicion; at the unconscious level, the good faith of the social bond is preserved by being alienated in money, in something that cannot lie—something that is dead. Yet the same argument will inevitably be applied to money itself; there is no way of freeing oneself from this new version of Gresham's Law. There is no way of stopping bad faith from pushing out good. As Bob Dylan puts it, "money doesn't talk, it swears,"[82] catching perfectly the ambiguity, embodied in money, between speech as invocation of the dimension of faith and speech as reproach and indictment of the very possibility of good faith. Money, in its very nature, is potentially the yardstick of all other values; yet its very blankness reveals that it underpins everything else only because of its intricate relations with everything else. To specify one single and definite relation—to cocoa beans, to gold, to the Deutschmark, to the "instinctive confidence generated by use and years" that Walter Bagehot in 1873 described as the underpinning of the Bank of England[83]—is to make more visible, rather than less, the inevitable collapse of money. The rationality of the liar, the confidence-trickster, and the counterfeiter is at least available to inspection. The "rationality" of the truth-teller, the good citizen, and the banker is in its nature based on trust—"instinctive confidence"—rather than reason.

We are led inevitably to the conclusion that the psychopathology of the liar must be matched by a psychopathology of the truthteller. Ibsen's *The Enemy of the People* (also known as *The Public Enemy*) provides a classic example in its portrayal of Dr. Stockmann, a liberal scientist at the forefront of medical, scientific, and hygienic progress.[84] His discovery of hidden pollution in his town's water supply eventually precipitates his transformation from being a believer in the fusion of democratic, republican virtue with scientific truth into a scientific Cassandra and bitter elitist, a voice crying in the wilderness. Stockmann's decline is a parable of the beautiful soul: the scientist who, in acting in accordance with the soulless, objective, and eternal truth of science, can only find the moral disorder of the world outside himself, cannot see his own truths as implicated in the order of the good and the bad, as bound up with the cruelty and sympathy of his own society. He consistently fails to recognize that every one of his own actions—motivated purely, he believes, by fidelity to scientific truth—is *necessarily* interpreted by his fellow citizens—the liberal newspaper men, the established conservative cronies of the mayor, the petit-bourgeois moralizing householders and taxpayers—in accordance with their own self-interested codes of behavior.

Ibsen's portrait of Stockmann successfully evokes the tension between two incompatible value systems underpinning much of the sciences since the eighteenth century—neither of which Stockmann

35

will allow himself to recognize. On the one hand, there is the Enlightenment ideology of toleration and liberation, seen as necessary conditions both for the exercise of free inquiry and for a society of possessive individualism. On the other, there are the values of authority and domination, implicit in the reflex recourse to the hegemonic discourse of truth and the beneficent control of nature and society—values which cohered quite comfortably with the expansionist tendencies of Western societies in the nineteenth century. Proud to be a pariah in the name of truth, obliged by his high ideals to ruin his own family, Stockmann has now become a parody of the Nietzschean superman; his only position is one outside of society. His last line, his last lie perhaps, is that "the strongest man in the world is the man who stands most alone."[85]

Of course, the invisible microbial pollutants of the water are also the lies he is combating. Telling the truth about water: the figure of Dr. Stockmann is for us forever twinned with that of the mad American general in *Dr. Strangelove* who knows the truth about what the Commies are doing to our water ("Fluoride!"), and in the name of that truth unleashes the nuclear holocaust. But when Dr. Stockmann is restrained from voicing the scientific truth in public, he instead attacks the pollution and lies of civic life:

> I'm starting a revolution against the lie that truth and the majority go hand in hand. What sort of truths do the majority always rally round? Why, truths so stricken with age that they're practically decrepit! But when a truth's as old as that, gentlemen, it's well on the way to becoming a lie. [*Laughter and jeers.*] All right, don't believe me if you don't want to . . . but truths certainly aren't the tenacious old Methuselahs that some people think. As a general rule, an ordinary common-or-garden truth lives—let's say—seventeen or eighteen years . . . twenty at the outside. Rarely longer. But although those elderly truths are always shockingly scrawny, it isn't till then that the majority takes them up and recommends them to society as wholesome spiritual food. There isn't much nourishment in that sort of diet, I can assure you—and I'm speaking as a doctor! All these majority-truths are like last year's salt pork—like mouldy, rancid, half-cured ham! And that's

what's at the root of the moral scurvy that's rampaging through society.[86]

The truth of science, which derives its moral force from the language of vice and pollution, is silenced; in its place returns the public harangue of those racially inferior scum, his fellow citizens.

Admitting that there is a psychopathology of truth-telling, that there is as much, if not more, rhetoric at work in truth-telling as in lying, appears to play into the hands of the cynic who has little time for the high principles of the moralists. Lying is as old as speech, she would say, just as adultery is as old as marriage. How can one expect to draw a watertight distinction between the two, let alone get everyone to agree to it, when, as soon as your back is turned, the vow will be broken? The way of the world is that principles are useful insofar as they can then be sacrificed to expediency. As Adlai Stevenson put it: "A lie is an abomination unto the Lord and a very present help in trouble."

So: "everyone lies." But is this necessary, or is it just a weakness which moral reform could hope to rectify? In his "Everyone Has to Lie,"[87] Harvey Sacks wonders whether this statement, and others like it that crop up in everyday conversation, is true or false. Specifically, he proposes that finding "cases" for which the statement does not apply is not an appropriate way of evaluating the truth or falsity of such conversational statements. He thus shifts the question from "Is this true or false?" to "Under what conditions is the question 'is this true or false?' a legitimate, or even comprehensible, one?"[88] Sacks notes, as Austin had done before him, that a more fundamental criterion, and one that has to be settled before truth/falsity is raised, let alone decided, is whether a statement is serious or a joke. We can, and should, multiply these criteria:[89] we have to decide whether the person who makes the statement is acting or not, whether he is intent on giving pleasure or not, whether he is being childish or not, and so forth.[90] Sacks's solution is as subversive as Derrida's insistence on the chronic undecidability that dogs all bipolar concepts such as truth/falsity. He proposes that the criterion for deciding whether "true/false" is a suitable criterion is the "sequential relevance": if a certain speech act is often followed by a true/false assignation (for instance, a complaint or excuse is followed by "That's true"), then one has a criterion of relevance of the true/false criterion. Since "Everyone has to lie" is often itself a complaint or an excuse, one sees that the true/false criterion is a response to a complaint or an excuse.

This criterion may seem overly legalistic in its nature: after all, law courts are supposedly the institution in society that, in the last resort, in the last instance, decides upon the validity of complaints or excuses. Sacks's criterion would make the legal model of truth the *only* standard of truth. It is important to be reminded that any society has a range of regimes of truth, ones that are almost certain to be mutually inconsistent. Nonetheless, we do not need much reminding that the most prestigious regimes of truth of modernity are those of the sciences and the philosophical doctrines linked with them.

---

Logic is not sterile. It engenders paradoxes.

Henri Poincaré

We might ask: What role can a sentence like "I always lie" have in human life? And here we can imagine a variety of things.

Ludwig Wittgenstein

Something peculiar happened in the course of the recent history of the notion of truth. It became commonplace to consider the business of "knowing things" and of truth as primarily a consequence of the properties of propositions couched in language. The propositional focus is by no means new, although it became, as a result of the "linguistic turn" of twentieth-century philosophy, a peculiarly comfortable one. Historically, the discourse of truth has been so saturated with the twin model of conformity with the real ("conformity with the facts, with the real"), and conformity with what exists in the mind ("having the intention to tell the truth, not to deceive") that the turn toward the proposition, as the site in which the real and the mental meet, has not entailed a revolution. Analyzing truth, then, necessarily involves a closer look at this propositional model of truth—the model that, for epistemological conservatives and radicals alike, has always followed Hobbes in saying:

> For *True* and *False* are attributes of Speech, not of Things. And where Speech is not, there is neither *Truth* nor *Falshood*. *Errour* there may be, as when we expect that which shall not be; or suspect what has not been: but in neither case can a man be charged with Untruth.[91]

Once it was established that truth can only be predicated of propositions, it somehow became accepted that the most important function of propositions was to have truth predicated of them.[92] And then a further step was taken: propositions *necessarily* possess a truth-value or function. The truth of a proposition became something like a necessary property, inhering in the proposition, rather than an accidental feature of it. Or to put it more plainly: the very *notion* of a well-formed proposition became inseparable from the question: is it true or false? In short, the narrowing-down process started by claiming: "Only propositions have truth-value," and then continued by claiming: "What makes a proposition of significance is the precise truth-value we can assign to it." To utter a proposition now came automatically to entail that one had made a truth-claim that could be examined according to canons of proof.

But scientists have not paid much attention to the excessive concern of philosophers with evaluating the truth-claims of propositions, despite the fact that the stylistic canons of their profession have made them paragons of epistemological virtue for many philosophers. Scientists, it should not be forgotten, conform to a pattern of discourse or rhetoric that is more concretely agonistic than this model has allowed for. Most scientists are more like commandos in the field, lawyers in a court, or entrepreneurs selling a new product than they are like generals at headquarters, judges on the appeal bench, or bank managers safeguarding the tally of accounts. To be sure, it certainly looks as if all statements in scientific publications are drafted with an eye to their truth being contested. However, not only do most of these statements never have to face such a challenge, but they are specifically designed to resist any simple confrontation of their content with whatever other features of the world (usually other propositions) are taken to constitute a test of their truth-value.[93] Given this, one might think that, even within science, the search for unambiguous means of ascertaining the truth-value of propositions is not only a blind alley, but also a red herring. What use can they possibly be?

Scientists may well be wise to spurn the imperatives of modern philosophy to focus on the truth-value of propositions—for reasons that philosophy itself has discovered. It is not only the poet who is mired in lies; that other great Western institution, logic, which is devoted to the analysis of the conditions under which truth is generated, also has to find its way around the question of lying.

One of the most striking instances of the fertility of logic is the Liar Paradox. Epimenides the Cretan asserts: "All Cretans are Liars." If he is telling the truth, then he is lying. If he is lying when he makes this statement, then we have an instance of lying that might seem both to refute the statement and to be an instance that exemplifies it.[94]

Logicians are quick to point out that lying is not what makes this paradox of such great interest and difficulty, although the formulation in terms of lying helps to dramatize the paradox and concentrate the mind on the deceptiveness of appearances, which is intrinsic to the very idea of paradox.[95] The family of paradoxes usually called the Liar can best be seen in the simple statement: "What I am now saying is false." The intention to deceive—the mark of the lie—is set aside. (Then we don't have to check out whether it is really Epimenides who is speaking, and not some Athenian actor masquerading as Epimenides.) Is a person who says "what I am now saying is false" intending to deceive? Somewhat wearily, we draw a line under the question by reflecting that the statement is confusing enough in itself without having to factor in the intention of the person who says it. A statement that is, on the face of it, true if it is false and false if it is true does not need any additional trickery from the intentions of the speaker to do its work; it has already played sufficient havoc with our expectations of consistency and truth-conditions.

What logicians do when faced with the internal contradiction of a paradox is to fix up our assumptions about the interpretation of the propositions involved. If, as Sainsbury argues, a paradox is "an apparently unacceptable conclusion derived by apparently acceptable reasoning from apparently acceptable premises,"[96] then the investigation of the paradoxes will inevitably lead to disappointment—disappointment in the deceptiveness of at least some kind of appearance. Disillusionment is thus the inevitable outcome of the work of logicians, no matter how firmly based are the new foundations for our methods of reasoning that they are attempting to establish.

The profundity of the Liar Paradox—as logicians persist in calling it, despite their universal agreement that the paradox has nothing to do with lying—is difficult to perceive. One may feel its force without sensing the questions that logicians have been obliged to address in order to escape it. One may feel its force acutely, as acutely as Bertrand Russell did, yet still feel, as he did in May 1901, that "it seemed unworthy for a grown man to spend his time on such trivialities, but what was I to do?"[97] It has often seemed sensible to run away from paradoxes, as if one agreed with Poincaré that logic is fertile but then rebuked him for failing to add that these progeny are all monsters. It is also a common feeling that this is not only a child's game but more specifically a boy's game. Brisk and blithe spirits, such as Karl Popper, have concluded that the only useful lesson to be had from the examination of logical paradoxes is that we should ignore them; but that attitude is the recommendation of someone who has been through the school of hard knocks that we know as logic. And it is a suitably paradoxical way of speaking, akin to Wittgenstein's famous ladder which he asks us to throw away after we have climbed it, to call that a useful lesson. The Liar Paradox was a ladder that Wittgenstein, in his later work, saw no reason whatsoever to start climbing: "If a man says 'I am lying' we say that it follows that he is not lying, from which it follows that he is lying and so on. Well, so what? You can go on like that until you are black in the face. Why not? It doesn't matter."[98]

"What I am now saying is false" still might be thought to involve the speaker's consciousness in the generation of the paradox. Nearly all logicians recognize the specific individuality of the speaker as superfluous to the setting up of the paradox; the paradox is only truly fertile in Poincaré's sense, of subverting our concept of truth, once we discard the speaker's intentions or her mark on the statement. So logicians prefer to clarify matters by eliminating—apparently—the speaker entirely:[99]

$L_1$.    $L_1$ is false.

This is the simplest version of all. If $L_1$ is true, it is false; and if it is false, it is true. But the reasoning used to arrive at these two conclusions is more exactly rendered as showing that "$L_1$ is neither true nor false"—and thus opens the way to questioning whether this is paradoxical. This clarification indicates that the sentence is only paradoxical if one assumes that every sentence is either true or false.

"The present King of France is bald" was Bertrand Russell's example of a sentence that is neither true nor false. The absence of any willingness to commit oneself to the truth or falsity of this sentence appears to stem from the fact that there is no present King of France in reality. There is nothing outside the sentence for it to hang on; our willingness to assert the truth of the sentence depends upon something outside of the sentence. "$L_1$ is false" chases its own tail too efficiently for it to get any grip on the truth.

Another relatively obvious approach to the paradox is to point out that the difficulties arise from self-reference: "I am lying" refers to the speaker referred to as "I"; the proposition "$L_1$.    $L_1$ is false" refers to itself. The clarification of Ramsey, Tarski, and others shows that the problem arises from the proposition predicating truth or falsity of itself, not simply from its *referring* to itself. Ramsey[100] distinguished between the semantic paradoxes, such as the Liar, which involve truth, and the logical paradoxes that do not, such as Russell's Paradox. Russell's Paradox—the class of all classes that are not members of themselves is a member of itself if and only if it is not a member of itself—certainly involves self-reference. But the problems with Ramsey's semantic paradoxes do not stem from self-reference, but from the fact that we expect it to be possible to say whether a proposition is true or false regardless of what its content is. When its content predicates truth or falsity of itself, this expectation leads us into generating a paradox.

The principal choice facing logicians, then, is to conceive of this slipperiness of $L_1$ either as stemming from its occupying a place in some logical space *between* truth and falsity, or as stemming from a failure of the sentence to obey a proper hierarchy of linguistic levels, in which the predicate that applies to all and only the true sentences of the language does not belong to that language. This predicate, the "truth" predicate, belongs to a language that is of a different "level." One can—indeed, logically, one must—then elaborate a potentially infinite series of levels of language, with the basic rule being that truth (or $T_n$) can only be predicated—without engendering the Liar Paradox—of a language of level $n - 1$. This latter solution, which was proposed by Tarski in 1937,[101] entails that the ordinary concept of truth of our natural language is incoherent. This leads to a restriction of classical logical principles.[102] Karl Popper interpreted Tarski as showing that no self-consistent language can include a statement concerning truth and falsity.[103]

What the two different lines of approach to the Liar Paradox—the indifference to truth/falsity approach and the hierarchy approach—both lead to is a retrenchment of the concept of truth. Truth can no longer declare itself. We envisage either a hierarchy of languages, none of which can declare propositions couched in them as true or

43

false; or we recognize that propositions are either true, false, or neither—in which case we might be tempted to think of truth and falsity as predicates that only contingently "happen" to propositions. This act of separation—of levels, or of predicates (truth$_1$, truth$_2$, . . . truth$_n$)—is common to all attempts to interpret the Liar Paradox. And we know that, in ordinary language, in the promiscuity of our everyday propositions, we will not achieve such a separation.[104] We will commingle our levels of truth, and may end up, willy-nilly, facing a paradox: a situation in which we have equally good reasons for believing one thing and for believing its opposite. "This statement is true" is not paradoxical in the same way that the Liar Paradox is, but it does open the same path to the difficulties with truth that the Liar Paradox does.[105]

Tarski also proved, in Gödel-like fashion, that not all true propositions can be proved.[106] Is the lesson we learn from the examination of the Liar Paradoxes, then, that we adopt a safety-first attitude to "truth"? That we take seriously the notion that propositions do not self-evidently declare themselves as candidates for truth or falsity—that the majority of them may have as their natural habitat that no man's land between truth and falsity? That we only invoke truth and falsity when the coast is clear—clear of any hint of self-reference, of a sentence proclaiming itself true, of a sentence referring to things that don't exist? If we adopt that strategy, we will have very great difficulties with sentences as simple as: "The Government has ceased covering up the truth about the prevalence of AIDS in the British beef herd." And what are we to make of "I am humble"? Are we to decide that "humble" is a predicate that can only be true of statements which do not include "I"—that there is something like a truth-reversal that goes on within the predicate "humble" when predicated of itself? Perhaps the lesson of the Liar Paradox is that we cannot expect anything to offer us a clear answer to the question "Is it true or not?"—not even logic.[107] There may even be room here for the suggestion of another subversive logician, Lewis Carroll, that there is nothing in the laws of logic that *obliges* one to draw a consequence, to *infer* the truth.[108]

There may well be other lessons to be learned. Bertrand Russell's solution to the paradox he discovered and thus to the Liar Paradox was the theory of logical types. This, the original hierarchical account which Tarski applied specifically to the predicate truth, was taken up by psychiatrists in collaboration with the anthropologist Gregory Bateson in the theory of the double-bind. The aim was to show how certain "propositions" or "predicates," if misplaced from their correct "level," will lead to forms of distorted communication. And, if these forms of distorted communication are situated in a context in which certain forms of inference are, in contrast to the playful logical world of Lewis Carroll, obligatory, then severe mental illness will result.

The theory applied to non-human communications as well: animals at play know how to distinguish between a "bite" and a "nip"— the playful "nip" is the form of communication that the physically identical but aggressive "bite" becomes when the animals play "a game." The notion of the separate levels of logical typing is thus converted into the notion of a game. The game is defined by the logical typing of the "predicates" or "acts." Communications within human families are then envisaged as obeying an (implicit) set of rules; when these rules allow for illicit predication from another game (another level of logical typing), subjects find themselves in a lived logical paradox. Their solution is the confusion of reality, as manifested in confusion of levels of language, which Bateson and his co-workers found to be characteristic of schizophrenia. One of the key elements in this logical machine for the production of schizophrenia is the injunction for the "player"—the chronically ill subject—not to leave the field, not to give up playing the game. This injunction is precisely what the playful Carroll reveals to be wanting in logic: the obligation to draw inferences. The basic paradoxical structure is given in the two contradictory communications: the subject understands that he will be punished if he loves his mother; he will be punished if he withdraws his love from his mother. And he is under considerable pressure, at the very least, to continue this communication game.[109]

The 1950s were the period when games became the deadly serious object and tool of inquiry. Wittgenstein transformed philosophy, conceived of as a patrician inquiry into language, truth, and logic, into a quasi-empirical and certainly workmanlike inquiry into the rules governing language-games. His worry over the Liar Paradox is thus a very different kind of difficulty from those of the early twentieth century preoccupations with logic and the formal languages of truth:

> Someone comes to people and says: "I always lie." They answer: "Well, in that case we can trust you!"—But could he mean what he said? Is there not a feeling of being incapable of saying something really true; let it be what it may?—
>
> "I always lie!"—Well, and what about that?—"It was a lie too!"—But in that case you don't always lie!—"No, it's all lies!"
>
> Perhaps we should say of this man that he doesn't mean the same thing as we do by "true" and by "lying." He means perhaps something like: What he says flickers; or nothing really comes from his heart.
>
> It might also be said: his "I always lie" was not really an assertion. It was rather an exclamation.
>
> And so it can be said: "If he was saying that sentence, not thought-lessly—then he must have meant the words in such-and-such a way, he cannot have meant them in the usual way"?[110]

Wittgenstein does attempt to get us to imagine what it would be like to be someone who lies all the time, even when he is asserting that "it's all lies!": nothing is steady or predictable, nothing comes from the heart. If he really did lie all the time, we would be on firm ground, it seems. The optimistic—or should we say overly trusting—analyst of the following problem certainly believes so.

> There is a guard beside one door which leads to Hell, another guard beside a second door, which leads to Paradise. One of the guards always tells the truth, the other always tells a lie. How, with one question, to only one of the guards, can one ascertain which is the correct door to take for eternal salvation?

46

The answer is: Ask one guard: "If I were to ask the other guard which door I should take to go to Paradise, which one would he tell me?" One then takes the other door from the one indicated.

Wittgenstein's liar seems to be mistaken about the meaning of words, or the rules of the language-game of lying: "lying is a language-game that will be learnt like any other."[111] But Wittgenstein's reflection starts with the assumption that one guard always lies, and then quickly goes on to consider what happens when the liar goes beyond a careful avoidance of the truth to the more challenging project of consistently misleading his audience. Wittgenstein soon sees that a liar who is reliable is not really a liar—he is as predictable as any utilitarian might wish him to be. But the liar worthy of the name will not always say the opposite of "the case"; on occasion he will tell the truth, and in so doing he will lead his hearer astray. The guard who sometimes lies is a much more formidable interlocutor than the guard who always lies. He will, in a word, bluff. We still understand what he is doing, but are less able to predict the outcome. The bluffer is still playing the game. Indeed, he thinks he has found a way to play the game better than the other players. Once the subject of the proposition—the speaking subject—knows that telling the truth may be a more effective deception than lying, we have left the Liar Paradox behind. Now, every proposition must be judged not according to its truth or falsity, but according to its function in the game of truth.

Lacan—and, as we will see, Freud—realized that the true liar may be bluffing even when he says "No, it's all lies!" And the unfortunate psychoanalyst of this deceiving subject may beam back to the patient the recognition that "in this *I am deceiving you,* what you are sending as message is what *I* express to you, and in doing so you are telling the truth."[112] Lacan separates the self-referring "I" into two elements: the subject of the proposition, the "I" as it occurs in the sentence, and the subject of the utterance, the "I" that utters the sentence. This subject of the utterance seems "prior to" the proposition: it is this subject that may deceive the other that is "beyond" the proposition by telling the truth, this subject that Freud's "skeptical" Jewish joke exposes:

> Two Jews met in a railway carriage at a station in Galicia. "Where are you going?" asked one. "To Cracow," was the answer. "What a liar you are!" broke out the other. "If you say you're going to Cracow, you want me to believe you're going to Lemberg. But I know that in fact you're going to Cracow. So why are you lying to me?"[113]

As Freud notes, such jokes point to a problem concerning truth: "Is it the truth if we describe things as they are without troubling to consider how our hearer will understand what we say? Or is it only jesuitical truth, and does not genuine truth consist in taking the hearer into account and giving him a faithful picture of our own knowledge?"[114] The subject that deceives by describing how things are—by saying "I am lying"—places the deception in the other, "beyond" the proposition. In this analysis of the Liar Paradox, the initial doubling of levels between utterer and subject points to the third party or term, "beyond" the strictly linguistic level—the third party that is "real." This subject knows that the other is well versed in the duplicity of deception and will repeat the fundamental duplicity, the doubling of the subject of the proposition and the utterance, in the act of understanding.[115] In so doing, the hearer will be duped. Or not, as the case may be.

One does have to play the game. Wittgenstein evokes the image of the perpetual liar in whose heart something fundamental flickers. We could give a different name to this person, by focusing on his lighter side: the bullshitter. Is this someone who has turned his attention entirely to giving pleasure rather than telling the truth, as if he were an Oscar Wilde determined to say *only* things that are *neither* true *nor* false? The bullshitter is nonchalant with regard to the truth; his speech is more like the idle speech of Heidegger, or like hot air, than it is like the dark and secretive lie. As Harry Frankfurt points out, "the essence of bullshit is not that it is *false* but that it is *phony*."[116] In order to qualify as a liar, one must be committed to the game of truth, be responding to the truth; the bullshitter rejects the authority of truth and opposes himself to it. Unlike the bullshitter, the liar does not ignore it. Of course, from the point of view of the truth, the bullshitter is thus a greater enemy of truth than is the liar. A guard who stood beside the gate to Paradise and bullshitted in response to any question would be the serious questioner's nightmare. What matters here is continuing to play the truth game.

Quite manifestly, the bluffer in a game of poker is still playing the game—he wants to win. (There is also a sense of bluffing, which I will leave to one side, in which a person bullshits in order just to get by.) The bluffing poker player plays the game in so committed a fashion that he has become the model player for modern game theory. The bluffer is to the game involving two players what the lie is to the single consciousness. Where the liar reveals the depth of a single consciousness, the bluff opens up the interaction of *two* thinking subjects, both engaged in the interplay of their own appearance and reality with that of the other. Once we know that the other player may be bluffing, we know that he is asking himself the question whether we are doing the same. The bluffer's bluff is not only about winning through being one step ahead, but also about preventing us from winning through being able to predict what he will do (that is, that he will not bluff).[117] The bluff in a game of two players creates the possibility of at least four strategies, not just three. It goes without saying that this must be a game in which bluffing is permitted; one might define logic as the truth game in which bluffing doesn't cut much ice. And the question arises: in which games is bluffing by all players—and hence the duplicity, the doubling of consciousness to which I'm drawing attention—permitted or forbidden?

The Liar Paradox—in the form of the sentence "There is no truth"—was used by Augustine to establish that truth is eternal. "Could truth not be eternal? If there was a time when truth was not, then there would still be the truth that no truth existed . . . and this

is impossible. Hence truth is eternal . . . and therefore God exists."[118]
This is one way to eliminate bluffing: establish the brute, unchanging
stupidity of truth. William Buckland acknowledged that the evidence
of the earth's history as written in rocks was preferable to the evidence as written by man, because rocks do not lie.[119] The scientist or
theologian aims to secure the unconscious stupidity of nature, so as
to eliminate the possibility that nature might be bluffing, might be
misleading us in the games of truth we play with her. Even the
disquieting experiments—both real and in thought—of micro-
physics, in which the position of an electron depends upon the
activity of the scientist, leading one to view the observer/observed
as one mutually interacting system, do not go so far as to suggest that
the electron is bluffing whenever the physicist turns up for work.

Norbert Wiener introduced a useful distinction based on these
considerations when reflecting on the kind of truth game we call
science. Having drawn attention, as I have done, to the pressing
problem of the deceiving God, the malicious God, of Cartesian
metaphysics and Einsteinian physics, he pointed out that the scientist
is obliged to regard nature as an "Augustinian" opponent in the game
of discovering the order of the universe. The Augustinian view
regards chance and evil as stemming from the imperfection or incom-
pleteness of the universe (including the human being in that universe). The opposed Manichean view regards chance and evil as the
work of a deliberately malicious intelligence or devil. The scientist
makes the crucial assumption that the forces of nature do not bluff;
he assumes that nature is Augustinian: "The devil [for instance,
Maxwell's demon] is not unlimited in his ability to deceive, and the
scientist who looks for a positive force determined to confuse us in
the universe which he is investigating is wasting his time. Nature
offers resistance to decoding, but it does not show ingenuity in finding
new and undecipherable methods for jamming our communication
with the outer world."[120]

In the playful Carrollian spirit of these scientists who, in the fertile
period extending from the mid-1930s to the mid-1950s, had realized

the scientific seriousness of games, Alan Turing proposed the test which now bears his name, and which still stands as one of the fundamental criteria by which we are able to decide whether a machine is intelligent or not. The test consists of the inquirer addressing questions to a concealed room, from which emanate replies, in the form of pieces of paper with writing on them. The inquirer must decide if the agent producing the replies to the questions addressed to it is a human being or a machine. If a machine concealed in the room can pass the Turing Test, it will have successfully passed itself off as a human being. It will, that is, have successfully *bluffed*—will have successfully pretended to be other than it is. The skeptics will still want to say that it isn't *really* a human being; that it's made up of wires, not tissue; that the machine's pretense isn't really a pretense because it is only running a software program and doesn't *know* that it is pretending. But the hinge of the test remains the possibility, for all the intents and purposes of its interlocutor, of a machine successfully pretending.

The ancient Greeks would have appreciated this witty and penetrating proposal of Turing's: the word "machine" is derived from a Greek root meaning "trickery" or "cunning," and the epithets derived from this root are often applied by Homer and others to Odysseus. Thus, to pass the Turing Test, the machine must reverse the semantic drift of the last two hundred years, through which "machine" came to mean stupid, unthinking, and mechanical, and thereby restore the original sense of wily, cunning, and tricky. The machine that passes the Turing Test does not demonstrate that it is a human being; instead, it "simulates"—that process which we increasingly regard as the privileged domain of the computer.

Wiener contrasted the "passive resistance of nature and the active resistance of an opponent," suggesting that this contrast helps us distinguish between the actions of the research scientist and those of the warrior or game player. "The scientist is disposed to regard his opponent as an honorable enemy. This attitude is necessary for his effectiveness as a scientist, but tends to make him the dupe of

51

unprincipled people."[121] Wiener no doubt had in mind Einstein's unworldly "flight from everyday life" with its search after "a sim-plified and lucid image of the world." What Wiener highlights is that the specific simplification the scientist demands of—and imposes upon—his opponent, the universe, is honesty. Now we are in a position to ask a far more challenging question: What happens to the procedures of science when they are confronted not by the honest universe, by a universe in which nature does not lie, in which there are no malicious demons, but by those Manichean beings, those masters of simulation we immediately recognize as machines who usually know how to pass the Turing Test and always do: human beings?

---

> By the time you say you're his,
> Shivering and sighing
> And he vows his passion is
> Infinite, undying—
> Lady, make note of this:
> One of you is lying.
>
> Dorothy Parker

> There is a great deal of hard lying in the world; especially among people whose characters are above suspicion.
>
> Benjamin Jowett

It is plausible to argue, as Einstein, Maxwell, and others did, that the motives for being a scientist include a desire to escape from a world of human intrigue and passion so as to enter a world in which neither nature nor culture, neither the fossils nor one's colleagues deceive. It is also plausible to see science in, and often enough since, the seven-teenth century as offering a discourse that is not subject to the disappointments and dangers of confrontation with religious or po-litical authority—as offering a free space of uncontroversial inquiry for gentlemen eager to avoid social controversy and conflict. However, even in that supposedly free space, it is not plausible to argue that scientists had effectively escaped from questions concerning trust in others and the authority of one's fellow man: "Every culture must put in place *some* solution to the problem of whom to trust and on what bases."[122]

Nonetheless, the field of scientific research on human beings poses questions about deception in both practice and theory, in relation to object and to colleague, that work on electrons or genes does not raise. Following Wiener's distinction, we can see that scientists who study human beings are trying to be Augustinians in a Manichean universe. And, confronted by deceiving objects of study, scientists readily turn to deception as a means of neutralizing this departure from their Augustinian ideal. It turns out that the endemic use of the deception of subjects in human scientific research is dominated by the possibility of deception in the inverse sense, the deceiving of the researcher by the subject: the deceptions in both directions have become intimately bound together.

Take one from the innumerable possible examples, one with important and obvious methodological consequences: the reason given by the early twentieth century anthropologist A. C. Haddon for rejecting as reliable sources for anthropology the reports of explorers, missionaries, and local officials: "How can you pretend to raise a science on such foundations, especially as the savage informants wish to please or mystify inquirers, or they answer at random or deliberately conceal their most sacred institutions, or have never paid any attention to their subject?"[123] The freedom of savage informants to lead inquiry up the garden path is absolutely determinant for the training of professional anthropologists. Their training in not being deceived is an endless one, and the source for endless professional in-jokes, gossip, and even crude accusations about "going native."

In other social scientific disciplines, with greater hopes of creating something more akin to experiments than any anthropologist committed to an ideal of noninterventionist "field work" would dare to entertain, the basic methodological procedures amount to systematic deception concerning the inquiry, precisely in order to circumvent

53

the threat of being deceived by the subject. Schematically, there are three rough categories of "behavioral research";[124] the first of these is experimental manipulation in order to create, induce, or provoke the effect that the experiment is intended to study. Such an experiment with humans nearly always consists in some kind of simulation, role playing, or deliberate staging. We are, as a consequence, in the territory of the Manichean scientist, of the game built on bluff. Probably the most famous such experiments, and ones that were certainly a landmark, were the Milgram experiments on authority.[125] Subject A was asked to instruct another person, Subject B, who was in reality an actor playing at being an experimental subject, to perform a task, and was asked to punish Subject B if he or she failed to perform the task adequately. The punishment consisted in giving Subject B electric shocks, which could vary from a mild 15 volts to a maximum of 450 volts, which the subject knew might cause death. Before the experiment began, Subject A was shown what a 45 volt shock actually felt like. In the experiment itself, the shock administered by Subject A to Subject B was not a real one, but the actors impersonating Subject B simulated receiving the shocks.

Milgram found that a large proportion of his experimental subjects—Subject A's—would, sometimes on their own initiative, more often under subtle pressure from the experimenter, give very large shocks to Subject B's. They knew what they were doing, it seemed; they knew—or thought they knew—that they were administering potentially fatal shocks to the other subject. They also knew—or thought they knew—that the punishments were only part of an *experiment* about education and training.

It is not the inferences that Milgram drew from the experiments that interest us here. Much of the initial reception of Milgram's publication of these experiments responded to what he himself thought was interesting about them: what they revealed about the extent to which ordinary people can be led into inflicting cruel punishments upon other ordinary people once they are placed in a situation in which they simply follow the orders of a scientist in a white coat. For Milgram, the immediate implications pointed toward the structure of authority in fascist regimes and toward the debates over the existence of an authoritarian personality—Milgram had initiated the experiments because of his interest in how the Nazi extermination of the Jews had been carried out. But it did not take long before Milgram's experiments became famous for a very different reason: not as the exemplar of the experimental study of obedience to authority, but as the exemplar of the questionable ethics of social scientists who engage in wholesale deception of their subjects.

Milgram had gone to considerable lengths in arranging for adequate "debriefing" of the subjects on completion of the experiment. He had preemptively explained that people are not suspiciously distrustful of and given to outguessing scientific authorities, and in fact the subjects had conceived of the experiment as a "psychiatric interview."[126] Despite this—because of this—Margaret Mead noted, in her psychoanalytic vein, that "when such a subject is debriefed, he can accept such debriefing only by some other ruse, such as in the identification with the lying experimenter or in the decision that social science is a bunch of confidence tricks and now he also knows a few."[127] Milgram's experiments had become an education in deception, rather than in obedience to authority, and formed one of the principal instances upon which new and rigorously binding ethical codes for social science research were developed in the 1970s, particularly in the United States.[128] Having initially been read as revealing the seamy, unpalatable side of human beings in general, the experiments were now taken to reveal the seamy, unpalatable side of certain human beings in particular: those who experiment on human beings. The double claim to fame of these experiments reveals a fundamental tension in the aims of the social sciences. Having been admired as a shining example of what social scientific experimentation should be, with beautifully designed experiments employing skillful deception of the subjects, they became a shining example of what social science experimentation should *never* be, precisely because of the deception of those subjects. Milgram's very success in preemptively deceiving the experimental or observed subject so that he did not deceive the researcher (what value would we attach to the results obtained from a subject who knew that Subject B was an actor?) was also revealed as the central blind spot of the social sciences.

The second principal research strategy of the social sciences involves the questioning of respondents—through questionnaires, interviews, and other means. The honors here seem reasonably divided between the subject who lies to the questioner in accordance with his or her own private and unknown agenda and the questioner who systematically deceives the subject about the true topic of interest in the interview. The social scientist inevitably adopts that active attitude of questioning nature by reason and experiment—the attitude that Kant characterized as being not the passive attitude of the pupil but rather akin to the judge who "compels the witnesses to answer questions which he himself has formulated."[129] The model of the witness testifying to the court of reason is an inescapably seductive, and at the same time deceptive, one. For these witnesses, these interviewees, perjury will always be an attractive option. Someone like Margaret Mead, a skeptical critic of the interview methodology used by the Kinsey researches into human sexuality, and not herself noted for sexual austerity, could observe how these "physiologically-sophisticated" scientific researchers took a "professional pleasure" in discussing with self-conscious honesty "the rather limited details of their sexual lives," but "became particularly angry if more sophisticated social scientists suggested that some of the respondents to the Kinsey questionnaire had lied."[130] Whichever way, for the court of the social sciences, deception may well be the rule, and certainly not the exception.

The third strategy, participant observation, revives Haddon's worries about the reliability of informants, but also calls forth the realization of the necessary disguise that the participant-observer must assume. The flavor of these debates—and the place of disguise in them—can be gauged from the reply of another controversial social scientist, Laud Humphreys, to criticism of his participant-observer study of anonymous homosexual rendezvous in public places: "The wonder to me is not that some sociologist might endanger his ethical integrity and that of his profession by standing around in public lavatories making mental notes on the art of fellatio . . . Concern about 'professional integrity,' it seems to me, is symptomatic of a dying discipline. Let the clergy worry about keeping their cassocks clean; the scientist has too great a responsibility for such compulsions!"[131]

Within the most sophisticated of the participant-observation traditions, that of ethnomethodology, the problem of deception is overcome by accepting it wholeheartedly.[132] Social actors are seen as possessing a repertoire of roles; social life is simply the process of "carrying on" within the framework of implicit and efficacious conventions embodied in social action. Being an ethnomethodologist is just one more role, in accordance with another, not particularly remarkable, set of repertoires known as social science. Endorsing wholeheartedly a rigorous agnosticism about inner lives, intentionality, and so forth, the ethnomethodologist experiments with repertoires, just as actors experiment with roles—introducing a touch of Beckett into Shakespeare. The theory of the social actor is precisely that paradoxical theory of the actor spelled out by Diderot in his *Paradoxe sur le comédien*. Is the actor acting most perfectly when he is pure simulation, going through the motions in a most artful and controlled fashion, holding the character at a distance, exactly that distance at which the audience will experience him? Or is he at his best when he identifies entirely with the part he plays, feels all the emotions of the character, and *is* that character, to all intents and purposes save one—that he is only acting? As in the forays of one of the most famous of all participant-observers, Erving Goffman, or in the deception of the ethnomethodologist in his experiments that breach social order in order to reveal what rules govern that order, or in his masquerading as stupid in order to get scientists to tell him what exactly they are up to—all these performances are just supplementary but unexceptional elements of deception in a social life whose very existence is predicated on the dialectic of the mask and the hidden.

The ethnomethodological approach allows the question of the truth or lies told to the observer (or "participant understander") by the observed subject (or, as the understander would prefer to describe him in Goffmanesque mode, "actor" or "native friend") to be defused in a manner akin to the psychoanalytic. The understander does not have to know whether he is being told lies or the truth (as the friend sees it), since he only wishes to know what counts as an "account" within that subculture. "A lot can be learned even if respondents regularly tell lies!" writes Harry Collins, his exclamation mark indicating that he knows full well he is on territory that is very sensitive for the social scientist: "questions of individual motive are entirely beside the point. The same would apply if an actor were giving a false account of his own actions. The fact that the false account is what *could* be a correct account in that society is enough. A false account is therefore as meaningful as a correct account. The fact that it could be a plausible lie in that society is the crucial point. Without understanding, it is no more possible to give an inaccurate account, or to tell a lie, than it is to tell the truth."[133] This methodological principle is, as we shall see, similar to the psychoanalytic premises concerning the patient's speech; but, beyond revealing the specific discursive structure of the plausible, it does not explore the complex internal relations that might exist between truth and lies.

In all three of these principal research strategies, the researcher is tempted into deceiving the subject in order to render her unconscious of the true nature of the observer's interest. The social psychologist hopes to *forestall* the possibility of the subject of the experiment deceiving the experimenter, either by insisting that the experimental subject be completely naive and innocent of the experimenter's goals, or by placing her in a situation in which she has, according to the experimenter, minimal motive for such deception—often enough by making the experiment boring and confusing. The test for the necessity of deception in social scientific inquiry should always be: why doesn't the experimenter perform the experiment on himself? If the principal reason for not doing so is the impossibility of finding out what he wishes to find out if the object of knowledge *knows* that there is such a project of finding out afoot, then deception is necessary.

The psychoanalytic procedure is the exact opposite on this point. If we consider psychoanalysis as belonging to the social sciences, we will be tempted to cast the analyst as the researcher. But if there is something that the experimenter—the analyst—cannot find out by self-analysis, then it doesn't count as psychoanalytic knowledge. In this comparison of psychoanalysis and the other social sciences another exact inversion exists: the experimental subject is often paid to participate in experiments, whereas the psychoanalytic subject will pay the psychoanalyst. This little financial detail is not without its significance. The knowledge engendered by psychoanalysis is subject to the supposed laws of equality, evenhandedness, and "trust" embodied in contractual relations, whereas the academic psychologist, through the introduction of the financing third party (whether grant or institution), introduces relations of authority and power, the vertical chain of command that relations of responsibility as opposed to honor bring with them.[134]

---

It is more shameful to mistrust one's friends than to be fooled by them.

La Rochefoucauld

If psychoanalysis can be considered under the rubric of the social sciences, it has at least an equal claim to belong to the world of medicine. And, despite the interest of the debates over deception in the social sciences, more may be learned about the psychoanalyst's strategy if we compare suggestion and its analytic sibling, transference, with the most universal of all the deceptions practiced on subjects by human scientists: the placebo. This evergreen standby of the doctor has more recently also become the essential ally, not to say the principal alibi, of medical research. The placebo is interesting not least because it reveals the extent to which medicine also inevitably struggles with the questions of deception endemic to the human sciences, thus suggesting that medicine should, in all fairness, be regarded, together with law, as the oldest and most sophisticated of the human sciences.

The placebo effect has been defined as what every medical treatment has in common.[135] Expanding this recognition into an inquiry concerning what doctors and patients are doing with one another led Michael Balint to propose that the "drug doctor" is the principal mode of treatment available to all forms of medical treatment. As we will see, gauging the placebo effect is a difficult task—it is, like hysteria, a joker in the medical bag of tricks, a truly protean imponderable in the field of medical therapeutics. Precisely that protean, tricky character is what makes it both interesting and valuable. Recently, attention has been paid to it for at least three different reasons.

First, the placebo effect is the shame of a scientific medicine, since its effective use requires that the patient be kept in the dark about what is being done to him, and the most reliable form of the placebo effect would require the doctor or the medical profession as a whole also being kept in the dark. Given what has been said about the relation between science and deception, it is clear that the placebo effect will, in a medical culture dominated by experimental science, never be welcomed with naively open arms.

Second, the placebo is used as the baseline against which to test the claims of experimental scientific medicine. Ever since the double blind clinical trial became established in the 1950s and 1960s as the authorized method of testing the claims of new—and old—forms of treatment, the placebo has become the negative touchstone of all medical treatment.

Finally, the placebo effect is the focus of more recent concerns about the ethics of medical treatment, precisely because it necessitates deception. Note that this third concern is quite distinct from the first, which expresses an epistemological anxiety. Here the concern is ethical: it poses the question whether any form of medical treatment that necessarily involves deception of the patient can be right. The new bioethical philosophers, advisers to the medical profession, and ethics committee members are not the only ones who have brought about a reversal of a long tradition of medical paternalism, best summed up in L. J. Henderson's classic paper on the doctor-patient social relationship: "You can do harm by the process that is quaintly called telling the truth. You can do harm by lying . . . But try to do as little harm as possible, not only in treatment with drugs, or with the knife, but also in treatment with words."[136] Since the 1960s, there has been an epidemic of veracity among doctors themselves: according to a survey, in 1961 88 percent of American doctors avoided informing patients of a diagnosis of cancer, whereas in 1979 98 percent had at least a policy—so they said—of telling patients.[137] Telling patients the truth is the doctor's part in the new doctrine of "informed consent," as it was christened by a Kansas judge in 1960. This doctrine has swept all before it, bringing in its train complex legal trials and arguments, new professional advisers and offices in medical centers, and committees to advise on complex medical decisions. The bureaucracy of veracity now weighs heavily on the medical profession. The compulsion to openness, to public honesty and accountability, has become virtually impossible to resist, not least because of the policing functions of the media. "The whole moral structure of our time rests on the Eleventh Commandment, 'Thou shalt not lie!'; and the journalist came to realize that thanks to a mysterious provision of history, he is to become its administrator."[138]

How far does the placebo, the epitome of deception in the best interests of the other, resist the new veracity? What are the consequences of accepting not only that lying is the oil of the wheels of society, but that the specific medical form of lying might have an essential function in securing the aims of medicine?

The general split between truth and lies is neatly reduplicated in the division between the scientific cure, which aims at specificity, and the placebo, which is inherently general—so general, in fact, that the doctor can never be sure what elements contribute to the effect. We are used to thinking of the placebo as a pill: the sugar pill or, often enough, a low-grade drug prescribed so that the doctor will believe in the treatment as well (studies show that the doctor's belief in the placebo improves its success rate).[139] From the doctor's point of view, a sensible definition is the following: "a form of medical therapy, or an intervention designed to simulate medical therapy, that is believed to be without specific activity for the condition being treated and that is used . . . for its symbolic effect."[140] But the placebo effect must be seen as much more than the pill or a symbolic gift: it must include the visit to the doctor, the ambiance of the clinic or doctor's office, the way in which the doctor negotiates the encounter, the little signs of bodily consolation offered, the confidence and understanding that the doctor can draw upon, especially if the doctor and patient have a long collective history of medical encounters both urgent and mundane.

In this sense, the placebo is the technological fix that answers Houston's question: "How can the doctor himself, as a therapeutic agent, be refined and polished to make of him a more potent agent?"[141]—a question that dates from 1938, the heyday of medical paternalism and medicine's respect for psychoanalytic visions of the doctor. In today's environment, we could reconceive the placebo effect as being whatever in the patient's relationship to the doctor, to his institutions, and to the medical profession sustains the project of the cure. Thus the availability of sophisticated technological medicine may offer more rather than fewer opportunities for the placebo effect to take hold, since the diagnostic process itself—the more high-tech the better—may now do what the sugar pill used to.[142] Thus we are required to consider what might make a medical culture—for instance, high-tech medicine in the 1990s, universal health insurance of the 1960s in Europe, or nihilistic Western medicine of the late nineteenth century—more or less "placebogenic," to coin a term.

How effective can the placebo effect be? The available data are ambiguous and often enough contradictory; but some indication can be had from the following brief overview. Many studies show placebos to have an effect on between 30 and 40 percent of cases. When used in a double blind trial alongside a supposedly active drug, the placebo effect may be as high as 50 or 60 percent, whereas the active drug has an effect in 70 percent of cases—and such a rate would be deemed quite satisfactory by the researchers; the comparable rates after two weeks of treatment might be 37 percent and 56 percent. Alongside these rough and possibly unreliable figures one must place the recognition that the placebo effect is the most reliable and tested part of medicine: "unlike most other forms of therapy, the placebo effect has withstood the test of time and continues to be safe and inexpensive,"[143] writes Spiro apropos of a famous series of placebo operations—the surgical ligation of the internal mammary artery.[144] The therapeutic effect of all coronary bypass surgery, developed since the early 1960s, includes a major placebo component, since improvement occurs even when grafts do not function.[145] A recent study showed that treatment of asthma, ulcers, and herpes simplex has a placebo efficacy as high as 66 percent.[146] And it should be noted that the drugs implicated in such treatments are among the greatest money spinners of modern pharmaceutical medicine: Zantac (ulcers) and Zovirax (herpes) are two of the five highest-selling drugs on the world legal drug market in the 1990s.

What conclusions are we to draw? Should we say that the active drug is 1.3 times better than the placebo? Or should we boldly conclude that the "active" or "specific" drug is only a third as active as the "general" placebo, since as much as 70 percent of its effect must be attributed to the placebo? The difficulty of interpreting such figures is compounded by the fact that the populations under test are not entirely random: researchers often weed out at a preliminary stage patients who they judge are particularly prone to the placebo effect.[147] Thus these are, if anything, rather conservative estimates of the placebo effect's overall score throughout a population.

One safe conclusion to be drawn is the following: it will always be preferable to combine the placebo effect with any active drug that is administered, since their combined activity is greater than either individually. To put the point more forcefully so that its extensive consequences can be properly seen: any medical practice that militated *against* the placebo effect in favor of the active component of a treatment would be very likely to have an overall deleterious effect on the patient's chances of improving. This point translates the basic recognition that the placebo effect is the traditional backbone of all medical treatments: it is what they all have in common. It is, simply put, what makes them treatments. And an estimate of its efficacy very rarely falls below 35 percent.

These figures make the placebo effect seem clear and uncontroversial, unless one has other reasons for distrusting this particular medical technology. Things, however, are not so simple. First, placebos have very little effect on many identifiable organic or structural diseases; they may bring substantial relief from the pain and suffering associated with these diseases, but they do not fundamentally affect such identifiable disease states. Exactly what proportion of all disease states are "pain and suffering," "illness" as opposed to disease, to use Spiro's terms; exactly what proportion are psychological or psychosomatic; exactly what proportion are stubborn, chronic illnesses that doctors persistently fail to find the cause of—and exactly what proportion of these categories, which may or may not collapse into one another, are eminently susceptible to the variety of placebo effects on offer—these questions are difficult to answer. Is it 80 percent, as Spiro estimates, talking of pain and suffering? Is it the 47 percent that Cabot estimated in 1907, or the 84 percent whose principal motive for coming to the Massachussetts General Hospital in 1964 was psychological distress?[148] Or the rough and ready two-thirds that Michael Balint estimated as the normal proportion of patients on an English GP's caseload who could be said to have conditions that were largely psychological or neurotic in character?

Second, the placebo effect shows wide variation, both from country to country and from region to region: in one study, the efficacy of placebos ranged from 20 percent in London and 50–60 percent in the United States to 70 percent in Switzerland; in another, from 44 percent in London to 73 percent in Dundee. The unpredictable variation in the placebo effect is much greater than with active drugs, although it is not clear that one particular effect seen with active drugs, the fashionable effect, holds good for the placebo: "At first, in uncontrolled trials drug therapy for angina usually proves effective in 60 to 70 percent of patients, but gradually the number of people helped by a new drug diminishes to a 30 or 40 percent 'placebo effectiveness.'"[149] What determines these wide variations? The answers are speculative: cultural, economic, and similar factors may vary from population to population, as may the techniques and beliefs of the doctors.

This mysterious variability in the placebo effect may well stem from the bond between the doctor and patient. And it is precisely this bond that the use of placebos in clinical research trials is intended to eliminate as a variable. This may or it may not mean that it is permanently destroyed.[150] But, from the point of view of the scientific research study, the index of perfect success would amount to its permanent elimination: finding an active drug that had a uniquely specific, 100 percent success rate under all circumstances, irrespective of medical context and history. This ideal is a goal that governs the unfolding of the research project, whether or not the active drug is 100 percent successful or is less successful than the placebo—as in the double blind trial of internal mammary artery ligation, where 100 percent of the cohort of patients who underwent simple incision under a local anesthetic showed considerable improvement in their angina, compared with the cohort that actually had the ligation performed on them, of whom only 76 percent reported the same improvement.[151]

In nearly all research trials, the patient is informed that, if she consents, she will be given either an active drug or an inactive drug or treatment.[152] This raises what appears to be an ethical question: is it ever possible "to get from a patient with an acute illness valid informed consent to any kind of randomized therapeutic trial"?[153] This may appear to be exclusively an ethical issue, stemming from the anxiety and distortions of perception and belief that develop from the patient's relationship to acute illness. But it is intimately bound up with a question about what is actually taking place in a clinical trial: the patient is asked to consent to being the subject of a scientific experiment which also includes within itself a chance, a lottery chance, of being given something that will cure her illness. Thus the patient is asked to consent to two things at once: being a scientific subject and being a medical patient, without the possibility of being able to consent to one without the other. Could this ever be valid informed consent? What is clear to the patient is that her medical relationship to the doctor (or doctors) has been compromised or annulled by her incorporation into a scientific research study.

In his book *The Doctor, His Patient, and the Illness*, Michael Balint coined the term "collusion of anonymity" to describe the process by which a patient with a mysterious set of symptoms is referred—together with his case notes—for tests from one doctor to another, from one hospital department to another, from one specialist hospital to another, until, often enough, he arrives back with his general practitioner with a sheaf of results indicating that "the specialists" could find nothing specific in or "special" about the patient. No one has taken responsibility for the patient; no one has entered into the process of negotiation and promising that constitutes the basic business of medical consultation. In the process, the patient has become dispirited, distrustful of doctors, and skeptical of any possible cure. The joint stock of the ongoing therapeutic relationship has been largely spent.

The randomized clinical trial is another efficient way of getting rid of this capital; it too depends upon anonymity, since neither doctor nor patient knows what is happening between them, responsibility for the treatment having been ceded to the scientific researchers in charge of the randomization procedure. The placebo effect—the constitutive lie of the medical relationship—has thus been abused to the point of self-destruction.

In the process, the connection between trust, promising, and the lie (the placebo) is revealed to be very different from the Kantian view that any deception undermines one's trust in the reliability of the other. Bok puts this argument forcefully, but in the exactly opposite direction from my argument: "The practice of giving placebos is wasteful of a very precious good: the trust on which so much in the medical relationship depends. The trust of those patients who find they have been duped is lost, sometimes irretrievably."[154] Surely it is the other way around: "the trust on which so much in the medical relationship depends" is not necessarily, or even very often, inductively founded on the experience of the success of medicine. To preserve and to exercise this trust, one needs to lie. Without placebos, there would be no grounds for trust that actually function as grounds—namely, the efficacy of medicine *without* science. Science, with its horror of deception in any form, functions perfectly well without medicine. The question is: can medicine function without the deception that is constitutive of its specific and overriding epistemological orientation, that of the cure?[155]

## II: Lying on the Couch

The loss of certainty of truth has ended in a new, entirely unprecedented zeal for truthfulness—as though man could afford to be a liar only so long as he was certain of the unchallengeable existence of truth and objective reality, which surely would survive and defeat all his lies.

Hannah Arendt

Psychoanalysis sets up the conditions for a scientific study of lies through a set of rules for the conduct of its discourse that speak to all the questions I have raised concerning the morality, epistemology, and everyday practice of lying. The context for the elaboration of an ad hoc but sophisticated epistemology of lying by psychoanalysis is to be found in the medical practices of the late nineteenth century. Hysteria presented nineteenth-century doctors with the possibility of a "disease" with variable, unpredictable symptoms—a disease in which the body deceived the doctor, led him on a wild goose chase.

As early as 1681, Sydenham had defined hysteria as "the condition of the mind in which organic disease of the nervous system is mimicked."[1] In addition, and often in consequence of this antiscientific possibility, it seemed probable that it was not the body but rather the mind of the patient that was lying—it was probable that the patient was a "hysterical malingerer." "The life of the hysteric is one perpetual lie,"[2] Falret wrote in 1866.

Rather than believe that nature could lie, could deliberately deceive and mislead by presenting false clues, clues that changed as soon as they were found, doctors attributed the cause of this protean entity to the patient's will. Hysteria highlighted the frustration of a doctor who believed he should deal only in bodies and observation when confronted with a patient whose variable symptoms might register a movement of deception. The hysteric highlighted the doctor's impotence in the face of a patient who would not name her or his pain in the correct way. The vindictiveness with which doctors often took revenge on these patients was seen in their frequent collusion with relatives' applications to courts to wrest away control of money and estates.[3]

The medical response to hysteria was twofold: first, an attempt to find a sure physiological index for when the patient was lying. The first lie detectors grew out of this preoccupation with the truth of the patient's pain, by reaffirming the veridicality of the body's clues: the polygraph, the galvanic skin response.[4] The measure of the equivocal success doctors and scientists had in this endeavor can be gauged from the later history of the polygraph. No extra-scientific institutions unequivocally accept the findings of the polygraph. The law courts accept the evidence of lie detectors with great misgiving and under highly restricted conditions; the restrictions are at their most lenient in the United States, whose institutions have traditionally been most open to scientifically grounded expert testimony. But it is evidence of the exemplary function that lies have in different regimes of truth that the first general rule to be introduced into U.S. courts concerning the admissibility of all scientific evidence was formulated to regulate the use of evidence from polygraphs. This rule, the so-called Frye Standard of 1923, is to this day[5] the principal criterion governing the admissibility of scientific evidence: the scientific technique, principle, or discovery "must be sufficiently established to have gained general acceptance in the particular field in which it belongs."[6] Underlying the courts' concern in this area was clearly the conviction that lying is too important to be left to the scientists, whose authority may sway juries too easily over this delicate issue. Given their head, scientists might have attempted to undercut entirely the distinction between lying and truth-telling in their search for Augustinian truths of the body.

Second, the doctor began to play the same game as his patient—began to deceive his patient through the art of hypnosis. Hypnosis had a double edge: on the one hand, it was intended as a means of securing total dominion over the patient's mind through control of the body and the suggesting away of pains and symptoms. Through hypnosis the tables would be turned, so that, instead of the patient deceiving the doctor, it would be the doctor who deceived the patient. But hypnosis was also intended as a sure physiological technique for the duplication and reproduction of hysterical symptoms, as in Charcot's work, which met the reproducibility requirement of science by using the theatrical techniques of rehearsal and staging: an unconventional if successful method of bringing human subjects under the sway of a physiological model in which nature cannot lie. But the theatrical model and the laboratory model may not be as far apart as one supposes; as Bruno Latour remarks: "If you think it miraculous that sheep which weren't vaccinated against anthrax died at Pouilly le Fort, or that Voyager II passes the rings of Saturn at the appointed hour, then you'll have to find it miraculous that Hamlet dies in the play's final scene."[7]

In contrast, psychoanalysis aims to be the science of lying inasmuch as it is the *only* science that does not find the prospect that the "object" of its inquiry may intentionally deceive the scientific investigator subversive of its pretensions to truth.[8] Casting aside the phobic medical attitude toward being deceived allows the analyst to accept as his or her primary focus those things the patient says that are most akin to methodical deviations from the truth: fantasies and dream-texts. The aplomb with which the analyst greets lies might be thought to be an expression, albeit an exceedingly rare one in both natural and social scientific discourses, of the "realism" or cynicism of psychoanalysis: it is founded on the expectation that the subject will, inevitably, being human, lie. The truth-saying properties of language are bracketed off as being idealizations—important, primal idealizations, in much the same way as are our idealizations of our parents, who, we unthinkingly assume, gave us this fickle and all-powerful tool.

In order to defuse the question of deception, which is so pressing for other human sciences, the psychoanalyst first of all places the patient in a situation in which she has minimal incentives *either* for telling the truth *or* for telling lies. Which way she goes is entirely up to her. The analyst is professionally disinterested in the difference between truth and lies. This attitude goes hand in hand with the highly idiosyncratic place of reality in psychoanalysis. The extent to which psychoanalysis takes no account of reality has perennially been seen as something of a scandal, but acutely so in the 1980s.[9] However, this particular practice, rather than being the quirk of a complacent bourgeois profession turning a blind eye to social reality, or of a family-centered idealism, bracing itself against the long waves of history, is embedded in the basic rules for the practice of psychoanalysis. This fundamental rule states: "Say whatever comes into your head, no matter how nonsensical, insulting, objectionable, or irrelevant." The rule thus implicitly excludes all normal criteria by which one judges whether a statement or utterance is pertinent, a faithful representation of reality, other- and goal-directed—whatever or whoever the other or the goal might be—or "serious."

Implicitly, the fundamental rule excludes all the criteria by which one decides "the truth." As Lacan puts it: "In analysis one lets go of all the moorings of the speaking relationship, one eschews courtesy, respect, and dutifulness towards the other . . . All our attempts and instructions have as their aim, at the moment when we free the subject's discourse, to deprive him of every possible genuine function of speech."[10] Although patients are asked to obey this rule—that is, they are asked to give up all the criteria by which speech is made sensible, is made to conform to the real, is uttered so as to entertain the other, and so forth—no patient ever succeeds in so doing. Individual patients are always sliding back into rhetorical modes they have been asked, and have agreed, to forgo: they attempt to persuade the analyst they are right, they attempt to seduce the analyst into believing in at least *something* (whether it is the cruelty of the government or the blissfulness of their childhood years), they try to coerce the analyst into distinguishing fiction from reality, jokes from the serious, dreams from nightmares. But the implicit requirement of the fundamental rule, and the attitude that the analyst in consequence adopts toward what the patient says, is that all these rhetorical ploys or varieties of speech act must be separated off from the other discourse the patient also engages in, the discourse that is in basic conformity with the fundamental rule. In other words, when the patient complains about the analyst's incompetence, she recognizes the speech act as a complaint; when the patient declares his admiration for the analyst's technique or taste in husbands, she hears it as a compliment. Analytic technique always requires the *separation off* of this aspect, this illocutionary force, of the utterance, so as to analyze it. Thus, for instance, Freud spelled out that when a patient expresses doubt about the content of a dream—"I'm not sure who the person was, it might have been the *au pair*"—the doubt is taken to be as much a part of the dream-content as the *au pair*.[11]

The radicality of this interpretive stance of the analyst is most clearly seen in his attitude toward negation—the integrity of which, after all, is the cornerstone of logical analyses of the truth or falsity of propositions: "'You ask who this person in the dream can be. It's *not* my mother.' We emend this to: 'So it *is* his mother.' In our interpretation, we take the liberty of disregarding the negation and of picking out the subject-matter alone of the association [*den reinen Inhalt des Einfalls*]."[12] The situation is similar for the affects, which include spite and self-righteousness as well as anger, fear, love, and hate: "the release of affect and the ideational content do not constitute the indissoluble organic unity which we are in the habit of treating them, but these two separate entities may be merely *soldered* together and can thus be detached from each other by analysis."[13] Hence the lack of interest the analyst displays in the question of whether something "really happened" is entirely a consequence of the interpretive technique of putting to one side certain rhetorical markers, bearers of illocutionary force, in utterances, whether they be claims as to honesty, urgency, importance, reality—or truth.

It is not so much that the analyst is *only* interested in fantasy, and *disregards* reality; rather, he is interested in *both* fantasy and reality, and disregards the distinction between the two. As Freud put it, in the letter marking this epistemological turning-point: "There are no indications of reality in the unconscious, so that it was impossible to distinguish between truth and fiction invested with affect."[14] "Impossible to distinguish between truth and fiction"—it is on the recognition of this "fact" about human beings that psychoanalysis is built. What distinguishes Freud's project, then, is that he recognized this "fact" *and* did not throw up his hands in despair (as he seemed tempted—but not that tempted[15]—to do). Freud discarded the idea that, as long as one concerns oneself solely with a patient's utterances, there exists a criterion by which one can distinguish the words as truth or fiction.

In the 1880s, when he was still principally practicing hypnosis, Freud conceived of his relations with the hypnotized patient as dependent for their efficacy on the freedom of choice with which they both entered into the "compact," as he called it.[16] It was this awareness of the freedom of choice underpinning the cure—and the implicit Enlightenment baggage of justice and equality that came with the freedom—that made it doubly ignominious for Freud to be forced, as he inevitably was, into the hearty reassurances and trivial deceptions which any slight setback in the process required of him. "The physician must constantly be on the look-out for a new starting-point for his suggestion, a new proof of his power, a new change in his hypnotizing procedure. For him too, who has, perhaps, internal doubts about success, this presents a great and in the end exhausting strain."[17] Indeed, Freud occasionally hinted that hypnotism could never be entirely satisfactory, precisely because the authority of the physician was fraudulent, and the entire success of the operation rested on deception:

> Whereas no patient ventures to be impatient if he has still not been cured after the twentieth electrical session or an equal number of bottles of mineral water, with hypnotic treatment both physician and patient grow tired far sooner, as a result of the contrast between the deliberately rosy colouring of the suggestions and the cheerless truth. Here too, intelligent patients can make it easier for the physician as soon as they have understood that in making suggestions he is, as it were, playing a part and that the more energetically he disputes their ailment the more advantage is to be expected for them.[18]

So, even when he was relying on suggestive (rather than rememorative) hypnotism in his practice, Freud's attitude was double: weary distrust of the deception it necessitated, a deception that both doctor and patient freely colluded in; and a belief that the playing of the parts assigned to them could bring success, so long as they were recognized as parts and were not subject to the exacting and fatiguing standards of truth.

Perhaps the playing of parts that was an important element in suggestive hypnotism encouraged Freud to avoid placing too much emphasis on the hysterical lie, as his colleagues were wont to do. In "The Aetiology of Hysteria" of 1896, Freud appeared to place himself in the position of mediator between the hysteric and his medical colleagues.[19] He certainly put distance between himself and his colleagues, inasmuch as he did not recognize their descriptions in the patients that he encountered. Freud never thought that the hysteric lies. Even in 1897, when he recognized that the stories told by his patients might not be of real events, there was no hint of the conclusion that hysterics had lied to him. Perhaps this absence was Charcot's true legacy to Freud: the absorption of the hysteric into the discourse of science had as its consequence the impossibility of describing the hysteric as a liar, since it was unthinkable to have a truly scientific object which lied. An unlikely trace of this attitude survives in Freud's intervention in a discussion at the Vienna Psychoanalytic Society in October 1910 of Adler's paper on hysterical lying: "The mendacity of hysterics calls to mind the old paradox of the Cretan: if a hysterical woman asserts that she has lied, it may be precisely this assertion that is a lie."[20] This acute passage is one more piece of evidence for thinking that Freud was more a philosopher than is apparent at first glance.

This dialectic of lying, deception, and truth was played out between doctor and patient in a malign form in hysterical malingering, in a more benign form within hypnotism, both against the background of a search for an ultimate truth of the disease. But within the very practice of hypnotism lay the recognition that fiction can cure as well as truth. And Freud was then led by his quest for the causal memory or mental event into the world of dreams, where he discovered, not that dreams were the opposite of reality, as had been conventionally supposed from Descartes on, but that, as with Russell's somewhat surreal proposition "The present King of France is bald," dreams transcended the distinction between reality and non-reality. He thus discarded the distinction between truth and fiction and created a new reality, which he called psychic reality, whose very principle of operation is fictionalizing (whether it be of reality, or of anything else). It makes no sense, Freud in this Wittgensteinian mode assumed,[21] to suspect a person recounting a dream to be deceiving or lacking in truthfulness. Dreams are the last place one would expect someone to lie and deceive—and that is why the lies and deception that emerge from a person's dreams are peculiarly valuable for finding out about the dreamer.

In retrospect, one can see that both the practice of hypnosis and its development within psychoanalysis were attempts to come to terms with the question of the utility of the patient's medical deception, one by cashing out the full utility of such deception in the only coin that counts in medicine, the cure; the other by defusing the question entirely, a piece of bomb disposal work that required an entirely new technology of conversation. The discourse of power and control which we in the late twentieth century more naturally associate with esoteric technologies such as transplant surgery, antibiotics, and bone replacement was first evident in the words uttered by the hypnotist doctor. We tend to forget that this enthusiasm for the cures made possible by hypnosis burst upon a medical establishment dominated by medical nihilism and therapeutic pessimism. One typical doctor, espousing the orthodoxy of medical minimalism at the end of the nineteenth century, envisaged a very different medical future from the one we inhabit:

> In some future day, it is certain that drugs and chemicals will form no part of a scientific therapy . . . The principal influence or relation of materia medica to the cure of bodily disease lies in the fact that drugs supply material upon which to rest the mind while other agencies are at work in eliminating disease from the system, and to the drug is frequently given the credit . . . Sugar of milk tablets of various colors and different flavors constitute a materia medica in practice that needs for temporary use only, morphin, codein, cocain, aconite and a laxative to make it complete.[22]

So it is worth quoting again Freud's strongest statement of the power the doctor could expect from hypnosis:

> Hypnotism endows the physician with an authority such as was probably never possessed by the priest or the miracle man, since it concentrates the subject's whole interest upon the figure of the physician; it does away with the autocratic power of the patient's mind which, as we have seen, interferes so capriciously with the influence of the mind

over the body, such as is normally to be observed only as an effect of the most powerful emotions.[23]

It is quite clear that Freud thought that hypnotism would allow the doctor to harness that general power of the mind over the body that we, with a somewhat impoverished vocabulary for such marvels, now call the placebo effect. Psychoanalysis would never equal these claims, as is evident from Freud's ironic recognition, some forty-two years later, that "I do not think our cures can compete with those of Lourdes. There are so many more people who believe in the miracles of the Blessed Virgin than in the existence of the unconscious."[24] From one perspective, the transposition from hypnosis to psychoanalysis was the transposition from the authoritarian, controlling ethos of Baconian science to the ethos of liberal-democratic Enlightenment science, the same journey that we saw Ibsen's Dr. Stockmann traversing in 1882 in the opposite direction to that of Freud in 1895. However, while Freud may have abandoned direct suggestion (the placebo effect), he never abandoned the view that large tracts of medicine employ the power of the mind over the body, whether overtly or covertly. His enthusiasm in the 1910s and 1920s for the work of Georg Groddeck, that exemplary doctor of the soul, is sufficient proof of that.

Historical controversies of the last fifteen years over the seduction theory have obscured the fact that the business of Freud gathering "data" about events in his patients' pasts was not a straightforwardly empirical one. Certainly Freud was in search of a single-factor causal account of the origin of neurotic disposition, and thought he had found it in the seductions or abuses of childhood. But the gathering of material from his patients was entirely dependent upon his therapeutic technique. In the period 1894–1897, the historical status of the trauma was undermined principally by the development of the twin pillars of resistance and transference in Freud's practice, which had immediate consequences for his attitude to those patients' narratives. Resistance entailed that the work of analysis did not take place in an atmosphere of agreement about reality or about the common starting-point of analyst and patient.

Then, by early 1895, with the recognition of the importance of transference, the question of the significance of the past compared with the present was raised. Freud found that the transference—the patient's thoughts and feelings about him, rather than about the past—intervened decisively and regularly in the course of the quest for historical reality:

> To begin with, I was greatly annoyed at this increase in my psycho-logical work, till I came to see that the whole process followed a law; and I then noticed, too, that transference of this kind brought about no great addition to what I had to do. For the patient the work remained the same: she had to overcome the distressing affect aroused by having been able to entertain such a wish even for a moment; and it seemed to make no difference to the success of the treatment whether she made this psychical repudiation the theme of her work in the historical instance or in the recent one connected with me.[25]

This account of the process of therapy predated the *enunciation,* let alone the discarding, of the seduction theory. Freud may well have adopted the principle of free association believing that, since nothing could be truly forgotten, it would eventually bring him close to the historical origin of the patient's illness; but it was the principle of free association that then led to the discovery of transference and thus to the undermining of the historical basis of his discovery. With the concepts of resistance and transference, both discussed in detail in 1895, Freud shifted the measure of the progress of analysis away from the historical excavation of the buried memories of the patient toward the work required of the analyst. Resistance was measured by the psychic exertion required of the analyst.[26] And the amount of work Freud had to do was exactly the same, whether he worked with memories or with transferred wishes and fears. Success was achieved whether patient and analyst worked with memories or with impulses in the here and now.

Thus, when Freud reflected that there are "no indications of reality in the unconscious," he was simply accepting on a theoretical level what the practice of transference interpretation already required: there are no indications of reality incorporated into the conversation between analyst and patient. The work is just as easily performed "in" the present or "on" the past—and what counts as real in the present (in contrast with the indeterminacy of the past) is guaranteed by the concept of transference. So, once Freud took his own practice as the basis for his theory, once he had brought his theory into line with his practice, he would *necessarily* discover that there are no indications of reality in the unconscious. It may be easier to see this if one substitutes into Freud's statement Lacan's definition of the unconscious as being "the discourse of the other": "There are no indications of reality in the discourse of the other."[27] There are no signs that accompany the speech of the other that reveal immediately that what she is saying is truth or lie.

What is *psychoanalytically* "real," what is unique to the reality constructed by psychoanalysis, is the transference—and everyone knows that this is a construct, an artifice, of the psychoanalytic situation.[28] To verify the transference by, say, the patient asking a parent if he *really* behaved like that toward his father when he was three years old, is to undo the very conditions that gave rise to the phenomenon in the first place—namely the thirst or demand for love, for the past, for knowledge, embodied in the very idea of addressing oneself to a psychoanalyst, rather than to one's parent.

Hence any call *on* the real in analysis is immediately seen primarily as a call which *occludes* the real. The apocalypse of the meeting with the real that an empiricist philosophy of science relies upon is only encountered by the psychoanalytic patient in a meeting with the real of the analyst—who, by definition, is not real in that sense for the purposes of the encounter.[29] The call on him or her to be real is rather like asking a jealous lover who has, like Proust's Marcel or Swann, constructed a world of knowledge by spying, by inferring, by investigating, to test that knowledge by confronting himself with the real of his loved one—an encounter that can never resolve the question which jealous knowledge is addressing.[30]

What Freud had given up was the deception that suggestion entailed. Having avoided in his early work the moral condemnation of malingering, he found in free association and the analyst's withholding of belief and unbelief a means of isolating his practice from the problem of lying and deception. Psychoanalysts following Freud were also, in the main, happy to ignore the problem; they talked of phantasy, not lies, thus indicating just how indifferent they were to the dimension of truth (and of lies). The consequence of the fundamental rule is that *all* modalities of discourse—whether it be the scientific regime of truth, the legal regime of truth, the dramatic regime in which disbelief is suspended so as to arrive at some "other" mode of truth, even the truths produced by psychoanalytic revelation itself— all these are grist to the mill of analysis.[31]

So the distinctive feature—both ethical and epistemological—of psychoanalysis was its *absolute* withholding of any moral condemnation of lying and deception in human relations, starting off with the analytic relation, which announces itself as being entirely indifferent to that distinction. Freud's willing suspension of disbelief in the moral certainties, both his own and those of other persons, entails that psychoanalysis always subordinates the discourse of blame to the discourse of discovery. As Lionel Trilling acutely notes: "But he did not blame them, he did not say they were lying—he willingly suspended his disbelief in their phantasies, which they themselves believed, and taught himself how to find the truth that was really in them. It is hard to know whether to describe this incident as a triumph of the scientific imagination and its method or as the moral triumph of an impatient and even censorious man in whom the intention of therapy and discovery was stronger than the impulse to blame."[32]

Indeed, the analytic relation is carefully constructed so as to eliminate all situations in which lying might be condemned. The obeying of the fundamental rule is both required *and* impossible. The money exchanged cannot lie: money never lies. What is equally significant, not turning up for the session when one has "promised," "committed" oneself to doing so, is not a subject for condemnation or reproach, since the analyst is paid anyway. From his side of the couch, the analyst refuses to open up the dimension of trust and faith, the dimension of promises and lies. The psychoanalytic contract is barren of all promises—of cure, of understanding, of love. Michael Balint wrote in the 1960s:

> The regressed patient expects his analyst to know more, and to be more powerful; if nothing else, the analyst is expected to promise, either explicitly or by his behavior, that he will help his patient out of the regression, or see the patient through it. Any such promise, even the slightest appearances of a tacit agreement towards it, will create very great difficulties, almost insurmountable obstacles, for the analytic work.[33]

Given that Balint was, as we have seen, also and contemporaneously with the writing of this passage, the theorist of the doctor as drug, the theorist of the doctor-patient relationship as one involving long-term trust and familiarity, we should place considerable weight on this extremely sharp division he draws between the medical relationship, designed to foster the placebo effect, and the psychoanalytic relationship, which can only prosper when all promises have been suspended *(aufgehoben)* for the duration. The analyst thus attempts to disavow the entire dimension of the placebo effect—of suggestion. The technique for doing so is simple: the analyst does not believe what the patient says—nor does she disbelieve. The "evenly suspended attention"—one way of portraying the analyst's frame of mind while listening and talking—is neither one thing nor the other. Hence from the start the analyst is excluded from being implicated in the patient's truth-functions and contracts.

The fact that the analyst is excluded from promises and trust, and thereby from being obliged to distinguish between truth and lies, reality and fantasy, does not mean that the discourse of analysis proceeds all on one monotonous level—quite the reverse. The patient still talks about truth and lies, reality and fantasy, even if the analyst does not. In particular, the patient may reveal a history of what he regards as lying, deception, and betrayal to which he has responded with guilt, self-reproach, or shame. If the patient informs the analyst that he is a "murderous traitor," she will want to know much more. But the last thing she will consider is reaching for the phone to call the police. Or so one would have thought.

---

> Moses did not include among God's Ten Commandments: "Thou shalt not lie!" That's no accident! Because the one who says, "Don't lie!" has first to say, "Answer!" and God did not give anyone the right to demand an answer from others. "Don't lie!" "Tell the truth!" are words which we must never say to another person in so far as we consider him our equal. Perhaps only God has the right, but He has no reason to resort to it since He knows everything and does not need our answers.
>
> Milan Kundera, *Immortality*

Freud treated lying as an everyday phenomenon, like slips of the tongue or dreams. Like jokes, which also have an involuntary effect on listeners, lies can be analyzed. One of the strong themes in his treatment of lying was the repudiation of the vindictive, accusatory attitude to children's lies. As he had done in his essay on civilized sexual morality, Freud took issue with those attitudes of adults which first treated childrens' lies as meaningless and then, in accordance with a double standard, punished them as signs of an incipient bad character. Of the 5-year-old little Hans, he observed: "The effrontery with which Hans related this phantasy [that his sister was with them the summer before her birth] and the countless extravagant lies with which he interwove it were anything but meaningless. All of this was intended as a revenge upon his father, against whom he harbored a grudge for having misled him with the stork fable. It was just as though he had meant to say: 'If you really thought I was as stupid as all that, and expected me to believe that the stork brought Hanna, then in return I expect *you* to accept *my* inventions as the truth.'"[34]

He thus portrayed little Hans as having discovered exactly those techniques of dissimulation that we saw Nietzsche ascribe to the weak individual employing his or her intellect in the struggle for existence—the techniques of irony and satire worthy of Jonathan Swift. Freud did not side with lies against truth, but he certainly did not collude with what he saw to be the hypocritical morality that endorses uniform conformity to a social ideal that is everywhere more honored in its breach than in its observance. At each turn, Freud would attempt to be evenhanded in the critical eye he turned on adults and children alike: "I do not share the view which is at present fashionable that assertions made by children are invariably arbitrary and untrustworthy. The arbitrary has no existence in mental life. The untrustworthiness of the assertions of children is due to the predominance of their imagination, just as the untrustworthiness of the assertions of grown-up people is due to the predominance of their prejudices. For the rest, even children do not lie without a reason, and on the whole they are more inclined to a love of truth than are their elders."[35]

In a short paper written in early 1913 entitled "Two Lies Told by Children," Freud underlined his view that the lies of children are often a response to the lies of adults, a kind of *tu quoque.* But, he went on, "a number of lies told by well-brought-up children have a particular significance and should cause those in charge of them to reflect rather than be angry. These lies occur under the influence of excessive feelings of love, and become momentous when they lead to a misunderstanding between the child and the person it loves."[36] He illustrated this thesis with two short case histories, derived from the analysis of two adult women patients. I will look first at the second case.

The lie this patient had told in her childhood consisted of bragging that "we have ice every day" to a school friend who had boasted of having "ice for dinner" even though she did not know what ice really meant. A second lie involved her use of a compass to draw a perfect circle in class one day, when they were supposed to be drawing freehand. She had refused to admit what she had done to the teacher who had discovered the marks of the compass on the paper, and who then consulted the girl's father about the lie and her sullen refusal to admit to it. Both lies derived, Freud said, from her strong attachment to the father she idealized, even though she could often enough perceive that his achievements in reality did not amount to very much. She boasted about him at every opportunity in order not to have to belittle him. "When, later on, she learned to translate ice for dinner by '*glace*' [ice cream], her self-reproaches about this reminiscence led her by an easy path into a pathological dread of pieces or splinters of glass [*Glas*]."[37] Her father had the gift of being able to draw circles freehand, so the second lie was a way of demonstrating what he, rather than she, could do—what she would do if she were he. "The sense of guilt that was attached to her excessive fondness for her father found its expression in connection with her attempted deception; an admission was impossible for the reason . . . [that] it would inevitably have been an admission of her hidden incestuous love."[38] The lie was thus a symptom in the service of her repressed love.

The first patient's childhood lies also revealed a story of unrequited love for a father. But their analysis was more complex, and also more revealing of Freud's technique.[39] The childhood lie that emerged in the analysis was also more significant than in the other case: once this woman had recovered the events in question from repression—or, putting it more cautiously, once she had recounted these events to Freud—she recognized them as the "turning-point in her life."[40]

The analysis of the events began with disturbances in the relationship between the patient and her analyst. She was not a resident of Vienna and thus was separated from her husband during the period of her analysis. The money he would send her would sometimes fail to arrive, and she would then be without ready cash. When, Freud wrote, he discovered this, "I made her promise that if it happened again she would borrow the small sum necessary from me. She promised to do so; but on the next occasion of financial embarrassment she did not keep her promise, but preferred to pawn her jewellery. She explained that she could not take money from me."[41] At another point during the treatment, she had taken to bringing Freud flowers, and he felt obliged to ask her not to bring them any more. This request threw the patient into a severe depression. All the discoveries of her analysis followed from their attempt at explaining this depression.

The patient recalled that, when she was seven, she had wanted to paint some eggs and had asked her father for money for the paint, which he had refused to give her. She had then stolen some change from him, but was found out. At her angry father's behest, she was punished by her mother. The punishment had left her inconsolable, and she recounted how she had then changed dramatically from being a wild, self-confident child to being shy and timid. Why had the punishment had this effect?

To the girl, being given money by her father so that she could then give him the painted eggs was her conception of love. The exchange of coins and gifts which her father had refused and for which he then punished her was modeled on an earlier event: when she was three, she had regularly gone with her nursemaid to the doctor's, where she had been given money to play with (and to buy her silence) while the nursemaid and the doctor made love. Ostentatiously she had played with the money at home, and her mother had noticed and inquired where the money came from. On learning the source, the mother immediately fired the nursemaid. The memory of this event had been revived and became causally efficacious four years later, when her father had refused to give her the money to buy colors for her Easter eggs. At that moment, under the influence of the revived memory of her nursemaid's transaction with the doctor, "taking money" had become synonymous with "physical surrender, an erotic relation"; thus her father's refusal to give her money meant that he refused her erotic satisfaction. "Her father's punishment was thus a rejection of the tenderness she was offering him—a humiliation—and so it broke her spirit."[42] When Freud refused the patient's flowers, already a repetition (in negative form) of her refusal to borrow the money he wanted to lend her, he was repeating her father's refusal of her love—hence her depression.

Freud's technique in this case clearly rested on the analysis of two significant disturbances in the analytic relationship, both brought on by *his* intervention in her conception of what counted as appropriate symbolic exchanges between analyst and patient. For her, to accept money from him was unthinkable—a reaction, Freud implied, to her equation of love and money. "When she was engaged to be married and her mother undertook the purchase of her furniture and her trousseau, she flew into a rage which was incomprehensible even to herself. She had a feeling that after all it was *her* money, and no one else ought to buy anything with it. As a young wife she was shy of asking her husband for any expenditure on her personal needs, and made an uncalled-for distinction between 'her' money and his."[43] Freud's gentlemanly behavior in getting her to promise to borrow money from him—somewhat unorthodox, the classical analysts would say—and his refusal of her flowers precipitated a wholesale disturbance of the system of ideas concerning love, money, and deception. Unpacking that disturbance revealed how her lie had been an expression of love, and how her father's punishment for it had been interpreted as a refusal of that love, thus marking her character, including the way she came to conceive of love and marriage.

Both these stories of childhood fibs turned out to be momentous because the person for whom the lie was told punished the child. The lie became a turning point in the child's development, or an ineradicable source of guilt and self-reproach. But the seriousness of the lie stemmed from the punitive attachment of the father to his ideal of veracity. In other words, the child suffers a trauma on account of the parent's superego; she internalizes the loved parent alongside a neurotic symptom or character-trait that has a lie at its core, preserved in aspic as a symbol of that superego. Grown to adulthood, the subject still refuses this superego—still refuses the punitive ideal of veracity. Instead of having her own superego punishing the lie, the child now become an adult has a symptom which expresses itself in other distortions, derivative of the primal lie. But the lie, it should be said, is pathogenic because of the moralistic attitude of the parent. The child thus falls ill of the parent's morality.

Take lies seriously, Freud implied—but not because of their being a first intimation of a propensity to sin or an antisocial disposition: "It would be a serious mistake to read into childish misdemeanors like these a prognosis of the development of a bad character."[44] Lies are an index of powerful propensities and passions. And, equally important, lies are an index of the conflict between civilization's morality, saturated with hypocrisies and protected by sanctions and sanctimony, and the powerful longings, both affectionate and domineering, of individuals.

During the First World War, the accent of Freud's critique fell most heavily on the lies of civilization. He portrayed the principal target of civilizations' prohibitions as being that cunning dissimulation that Nietzsche had credited to the individual, who, Freud wrote, "was above all forbidden to make use of the immense advantages to be gained by the practice of lying and deception in the competition with his fellow-men. The civilized states regarded these moral standards as the basis of their existence. They took serious steps if anyone ventured to tamper with them, and often declared it improper even to subject them to examination by a critical intelligence."[45] But it was now clear to Freud how hypocritical this demand on the individual was: "A belligerent state permits itself every such misdeed, every such act of violence, as would disgrace the individual. It makes use against the enemy not only of the accepted *ruses de guerre,* but of deliberate lying and deception as well—and to a degree which seems to exceed the usage of former wars."[46] And by the late 1920s, Freud's opinion of individuals had fallen to the same low level as that of civilization: "There are countless civilized people who would shrink from murder or incest but who do not deny themselves the satisfaction of their avarice, their aggressive urges or their sexual lusts, and who do not hesitate to injure other people by lies, fraud and calumny, so long as they can remain unpunished for it; and this, no doubt, has always been so through many ages of civilization."[47] What sounds as if it might become a moralizing criticism never does. The old man's identification with Moses did not extend to the introduction of new prohibitions. Quite the reverse.

———————

Have you ever told so much truth as when you were first in love? Have you ever seen the world so clearly? Love makes us see the truth, makes it our duty to tell the truth. Lying in bed: listen to the undertow of warning in that phrase. *Lying in bed, we tell the truth:* it sounds like a paradoxical sentence from a first-year philosophy primer. But it's more (and less) than that: a description of moral duty.

Julian Barnes, *A History of the World in 10½ Chapters*

I can imagine that to point out the existence of lying dreams of this kind, "obliging" dreams, will arouse a positive storm of helpless indignation in some readers who call themselves analysts. "What!" they will exclaim, "the unconscious, the real centre of our mental life, the part of us that is so much nearer the divine than our poor consciousness—it too can lie! Then how can we still build on the interpretations of analysis and the accuracy of our findings?" To which one must reply that the recognition of these lying dreams does not constitute any shattering novelty.

Freud, "The Psychogenesis of a Case of Homosexuality in a Woman"

Why is it, then, if psychoanalysis has a method that is tailor-made to avoid being undermined by the threat of lies and deception, that some psychoanalysts have reacted with almost phobic distrust to the possibility that the patient may be lying to them?

The fact that lying had been decisively sidelined as a problem for psychoanalysis is reflected in the overall paucity of attention paid to the malingerer, even to the psychiatric category that late nineteenth century doctors, sensitized to the sins of patients, had generated to capture baroque forms of it, *pseudologia fantastica*. A scattering of papers on the topic is all the psychoanalytic literature, both ancient and modern, can offer.[48] Certain of these papers do, however, reveal some interesting conceptual tensions surrounding the topic—they reveal that the problem of the reality of infantile scenes is intimately linked to the possibility of the patient lying to the analyst, and that whenever one topic is raised the other comes with it.

Sándor Ferenczi was Freud's foremost Hungarian disciple and intimate friend, who willingly accepted the epithet of the *enfant terrible* of psychoanalysis; he could equally well have been called the touchstone of psychoanalytic technique. More imaginative and enterprising in his experimentation with technique than any other analyst, Ferenczi came up with innovations ranging from his experiments with mediums and thought-transference to the active techniques of the period 1919–1924, in which he attempted to accelerate the analytic process by suppressing the defensive strategies and patterns of behavior that constituted resistance. The last phase of his experimentation with technique was to lead to his advocacy of a return to a version of the seduction theory that Freud had abandoned in 1897. Ferenczi came to think that, "having given due consideration to fantasy as a pathogenic factor, I have of late been forced more and more to deal with the pathogenic trauma itself. It became evident that this is far more rarely the result of a constitutional hypersensibility in children . . . than of really improper, unintelligent, capricious, tactless, or actually cruel treatment."[49]

This theme, the either/or of constitution versus trauma, of fantasy (as derivative of inner constitution) versus reality (what actually happened, as external event, in childhood), which had been set to one side by Freud, inevitably brought with it a revival of the importance of lying and truth-telling. But Ferenczi's formulations showed a strange tension. He continued: "Hysterical fantasies do not lie when they tell us that parents and other adults do indeed go to monstrous lengths in the passionate eroticism of their relation with children, while, on the other hand, when the innocent child responds to this half-unconscious play on the part of its elders the latter are inclined to think out [sic] severe punishments and threats which are altogether incomprehensible to him and have the shattering effects of a shock."[50] It is the *fantasies* that do not lie. Ferenczi does not discard infantile sexuality and the etiological significance of fantasy. It is not a question of *either* fantasy *or* reality for him, no more than it ever was for Freud. But he does revive the question of lying, both as regards the truth that patients speak and the attitude of the analyst to the patient, the fundamental attitude with which the analyst listens to the patient.

This final phase of Ferenczi's work was announced with a paper entitled "The Problem of the Termination of the Analysis," delivered in 1927. It opened with a case history "which some time ago caused me a great deal of concern. While dealing with a patient who, apart from certain neurotic difficulties, came to analysis chiefly because of certain abnormalities and peculiarities of his character, I suddenly discovered, incidentally after more than eight months, that he had been deceiving me the whole time in connexion with an important circumstance of a financial nature. At first this caused me the greatest embarrassment."[51] As in Freud's case of the woman patient who brought too many flowers to her analyst, this case begins to take shape in the transference—this time over the question of money, the medium of trust and fidelity that, for the purposes of psychoanalysis, is assumed not to lie. Ferenczi's analysis of the patient then proceeded to reveal his systematic mendacity.

Earlier in the analysis, the patient had failed to turn up for a session. The next day, Ferenczi asked him why he had failed to turn up. The man, rather astonished, insisted he had come. Ferenczi maintained that he hadn't been there. And, in his turn, the patient insisted that he had. Eventually Ferenczi managed to persuade him that he, the analyst, was right, that the patient in reality had not come to the session on the previous day. Not only that—the patient had forgotten everything else he had done that previous day. In the process of reconstructing what else he had or had not done on the previous day, partly by questioning others, a whole set of "illicit" activities came to light.

Once the lie about the financial matter emerged, Ferenczi con-

nected the two together. "When I obtained incontrovertible evidence
of his conscious mendacity I was convinced that the split personality,
at any rate in his case, was only the neurotic sign of his mendacity,
a kind of indirect confession of his character-defect."[52] But the case
provoked Ferenczi into the following reflections: "The fundamental
rule of analysis, on which the whole of our technique is built up,
calls for the true and complete communication by the patient of all
his ideas and associations. What, then, is one to do if the patient's
pathological condition consists precisely in mendacity? Should one
declare analysis to be unsuitable for dealing with such cases? I had
no intention of admitting such poverty on the part of our scientific
technique."[53] And Ferenczi made use of the shock of having been
deceived to draw up a new picture of psychoanalytic understanding.
"In an earlier paper I offered the suggestion that in infancy all
hysterical symptoms were produced as conscious fictional structures.
I recalled also that Freud used occasionally to tell us that it was
prognostically a favorable sign, a sign of approaching cure, if the
patient suddenly expressed the conviction that during the whole of
his illness he had really been only shamming."[54]

There were two different diagnostic signs, one the inverse of the
other, that Freud had noted pointed to changes in the relations of
the unconscious and the conscious taking place in the course of
analysis. The phenomenon Ferenczi was referring to, when a patient
suddenly decided that he had been pretending his illness, indicated
that the past intentionality, the meaning of the symptoms, was becoming available for the first time (since their inception), and, insofar
as the patient now felt that he was in intentional control of them—
could decide whether to have them or not—he decided that this had
always been the case. In the past, then, he must have been pretending,
in the sense of willing, to be ill. "I was (never) always ill" is the
proposition in question, where the *never* has been inserted as the sign
of the becoming conscious that has been achieved.

The other sentence that is a sign of an approaching cure or lifting
of repression is: "I didn't (ever) think of that." Freud's short paper

"Negation," from which I have already quoted, ends with the following passage: "In analysis we never discover a 'no' in the unconscious and that recognition of the unconscious on the part of the ego is expressed in a negative formula. There is no stronger evidence that we have been successful in our effort to uncover the unconscious than when the patient reacts to it with the words 'I didn't think that,' or 'I didn't (ever) think of that.'"[55] Freud's attention to the relation of negation to utterances makes it impossible for a patient to tell the truth, in the sense of making a declarative statement that corresponds to reality. The best he can manage is the declarative statement that affirms that reality in denying it. "'You ask who this person in the dream can be. It's *not* my mother.' We emend this to: 'So it *is* his mother.'"

These seemingly paradoxical sentences from a first-year philosophy primer are in reality the foundation of psychoanalytic understanding. "No" must be interpreted as "yes," precisely because some things have become impossible to affirm. Neurosis in retrospect, like love, always feels like a pretense. If that is the case, it makes no sense to place the patient in the spotlight that marks out truth from lies. Psychoanalysis as a practice begins when the bright light of truth is switched off; once the eyes have grown accustomed to the murk, making darkness visible becomes possible.

Laurence Horn's magisterial study *A Natural History of Negation* finds Freud's position here to be typical of what he calls the asymmetrical interpretation of negation, shared by Aristotle (sometimes), Plato, Bacon, Kant, Hegel, Russell (sometimes), and many others. This position regards negation as secondary to the primary propositional form of affirmation. Horn argues that this asymmetrical view is semantically implausible. However, he recognizes that in actual discourse, Wittgenstein's intuition is justified: "The feeling is as if the negation of a proposition had to make it [the proposition] true in a certain sense, in order to negate it."[56] The semantic interpretation, the refutation of the feeling, which is the position Horn endorses, is then given by Wittgenstein in parentheses: "(The assertion

of the negative proposition contains the proposition which is ne-
gated, but not the assertion of it.)" The interpretation is again tricky:
how does an assertion contain a non-assertion? How do we know
when propositions within asserted propositions are not asserted? Can
we legitimately draw the distinction between the mention of the
proposition and its use, between the mention of "the mother" and
her "use"? We are recognizably in the paradoxical territory of the
Liar Paradox. In a gesture similar to that of the logicians, Horn
concludes: "Like Freud's dreamer, for whom *It is not my mother* really
means 'It is my mother,' the strong Asymmetricalist thesis is literally
false but psychologically true."[57]

Let us return to Ferenczi's lying patient, and to the further reflections on the place of lies in psychoanalysis to which he prompted his
analyst.

> What in the light of morality and of the reality principle we call a lie,
> in the case of an infant and in terms of pathology we call fantasy . . .
> We had come to the conclusion that the laying bare of the fantasy,
> which could be said to possess a special kind of reality of its own
> (Freud called it a psychical reality), was sufficient for a cure, and that
> it was a secondary matter from the point of view of the success of the
> analysis how much of the fantasy content corresponded to reality, i.e.
> physical reality or the recollections of such reality. My experience had
> taught me something else. I had become convinced that no case of
> hysteria could be regarded as cleared up so long as a reconstruction,
> in the sense of a rigid separation of reality and fantasy, had not been
> carried out . . . One might generalize and say that a neurotic cannot
> be regarded as cured if he has not given up pleasure in unconscious
> fantasy, i.e. unconscious mendacity.[58]

Ferenczi was proposing that the intermingling of lie and fantasy that
is characteristic of psychoanalysis, whose object is psychical reality
and not material reality, has to be undone at the end of each analysis.
It has to be made clear what is fantasy (lie) and what is reality (truth).
To support this claim, Ferenczi pointed to the one characteristic that
those who have been thoroughly analyzed share, their "far sharper

severance between the world of fantasy and that of reality," which gives them "almost unlimited inner freedom and simultaneously a much surer grip in acting and making decisions."[59]

This new measure of the effect of analysis requires a new means: the honesty of the analyst. The patient relentlessly tests the analyst's dependability and good will toward him, probing mercilessly to catch the analyst out in an untruth or distortion.[60] Once he becomes convinced that the analyst is not lying, he can begin to test the possibility of doing without lies himself. The preoccupation with the honesty of the analyst and the reintroduction of the language of lies where psychoanalysts had previously spoken of fantasy developed into Ferenczi's final theory, in which infancy is beyond lies and the tenderness and honesty that children need are denied them by the eroticized and deceptive actions of adults in relation to them. Ferenczi proposed that the analyst walk a fine line between the principle of frustration that Freud had proposed, and the principle of indulgence with which he wished to supplement frustration. By indulgence Ferenczi was referring to Freud's own principle of freedom and tolerance that is everywhere to be found in parallel with his equally habitual severity: "Are not both these principles [of frustration and indulgence] inherent in the method of free association? On the one hand, the patient is compelled to confess disagreeable truths, but, on the other hand, he is permitted a freedom of speech and expression of his feelings such as is hardly possible in any other department of life."[61] Ferenczi could see the dangers of his own proposal, as he warned against the "errors of those who treat neurotics, not analytically, i.e. with complete sincerity, but with a simulation of severity or love."[62]

Recent discussions of Ferenczi's work have often contrasted him with Freud, as if Freud were identified with severity or its simulation and Ferenczi with love—or its simulation. Ferenczi, however, still saw sincerity as the highest virtue of all. Since, in his reading of psychoanalysis, sincerity is both the means and the telos of analysis, it therefore began to dominate his conception of the moral ethos of the analyst. It can be argued that Freud too, was a fervent upholder of

93

honesty, a seeming contradiction that is clarified if we make the distinction suggested by Adam Phillips between the Freudian (or Enlightenment) Freud and the post-Freudian Freud.[63] Take the following emphatic declaration: "Psycho-analytic treatment is founded on truthfulness. In this fact lies a great part of its educative effect and its ethical value. It is dangerous to depart from this foundation. Anyone who has become saturated in the analytic technique will no longer be able to make use of the lies and pretences which a doctor normally finds unavoidable; and if, with the best intentions, he does attempt to do so, he is very likely to betray himself. Since we demand strict truthfulness from our patients, we jeopardize our whole authority if we let ourselves be caught out by them in a departure from the truth."[64]

This has very much the tone of Ferenczi exhorting analysts to honesty in all things as a major tool for overcoming resistance. But whereas Ferenczi envisaged the honest analyst confronting the potentially evasive, lying, and defensive patient, Freud's paean of praise to honesty was elicited by a very different problem patient: the woman who falls in love with her analyst. Freud's exhortation to honesty is intended to stop analysts from falling into the laps, rather than the lies, of their patients. Some would say this figure of the passionate woman patient was Freud's weak point, others his strong point—certainly she was his sensitive point. The strong woman who would brook no opposition to the demands of her erotic life, who would tolerate no surrogates, who is accessible only "to the logic of soup, with dumplings for arguments"—this was Freud's exemplary patient.[65] The lying patient, in contrast, lost him no sleep at all.[66]

The note of alarm over lying sounded by Ferenczi, soon absorbed into a larger preoccupation with the distinction between reality and fantasy and the trustworthiness of the analyst as much as the patient, is heard again in contemporary psychoanalysts' writing about lying. "Can a liar be psychoanalysed?" asks Edna O'Shaugnessy in the *International Journal of Psycho-Analysis* in 1990, and, almost reluctantly, as if she herself is surprised by her own answer, concludes that he can:

Because a liar knows he lies, his lies are not cut off from the truth . . .
a lie is an acceptance of, and a perverse use of, a falsehood. I think this
is the origin of what we feared initially, that there is a deep antagonism
of perspective between a liar and a psychoanalyst . . . Nonetheless, the
lying [of the two patients discussed] was the means of communicating
urgently the fundamental truth about their early object relations . . .
The liar has to risk the abandonment of his present psychic structure
with an analyst whom . . . he will experience as a two-faced dissembler
. . . [The two lying patients] succeeded in getting me to take lies as
truth, so that I actually became a partner in a perversion of the analytic
relationship, unwittingly enacting it with them . . . If the fundamental
level of the lie can be understood, that a liar lies in identification with
a lying object, and, at the same time, if the patient's hostile lying, his
different perspective in regard to truth and also his perverse excite-
ment at using the lie to communicate with his analyst can be analyzed
in all their concreteness, I am sure at least of this: a genuine analytic
process can be set in train.[67]

The case histories O'Shaugnessy recounts are full of crises of
confidence in her own mental states and in the course of the analysis—doubts about what the real facts of her patient's life were, from
his false telephone number to his familial relations. The patient
taunts her with lies, she reflects, trying to provoke her into calling
him a liar and moralizing at him. "I had to struggle hard to hold an
analytic stance."

Surely, we reflect, such struggles and crises are the day-to-day
business of the modern analyst? Every analysis involves crises of
resistance, which may, if the patient is any good at getting involved
with other people, create a comparable countertransference crisis in
the other. Freud was particularly aware of how doubt and skepticism
were major features of such resistance: "'It would be all very fine,'
thinks the patient, often quite consciously, 'if I were obliged to believe
what the man says, but there is no question of that, and so long as
this is so I need change nothing.' Then, when one comes to close
quarters with the motives for this doubt, the fight with the resistances
breaks out in earnest."[68] Such resistances will involve the explicit
doubt and skepticism, which will not stop at polite questioning but

will inevitably become scorn, derision, belittling, ridicule, irony, not to mention abuse and the more complex strategies for making analysts feel confused and at fault. Particularly when working with the countertransference, the modern analyst spends his or her days being on emotional emergency call. The liar is just one variation on this theme—as O'Shaugnessy implicitly recognizes when she sees how to characterize him as exhibiting a particular form of a generalized narcissistic organization. What the lie does to the analytic communication thus may be no more—or no less—of a threat than the patient who disclaims all responsibility for what the analyst feels in response to his words, or the patient who systematically bores the analyst to tears, or provokes the analyst into making promises to the patient.

From the sheer rarity-value of Ferenczi's and O'Shaugnessy's cases it is clear how, in the history of psychoanalysis, the theme of lying gets covered over by the theme of fantasy.[69] Freud obviously had good reasons for giving up the language of truth and lies for a language less prone to misunderstanding. His replacement language, the language of repression, evades the insistence of intentionality and control over the other of lying, and it avoids the atmosphere of enforced intimacy that the language of truth and lies brings with it. But were the languages kept distinct? Didn't Freud often enough make it clear that repression was a form of self-deception—for instance, when he characterized repression as a "primary mechanism of defence, comparable to an attempt at flight" but "only a forerunner of the later-developed condemning judgement"[70]—the judgment that asserts a negation?

Certainly his theories have been understood by many, among them philosophers preoccupied by or sympathetic to his theories, from Sartre to Davidson, as concerned with varieties of self-deception. And wouldn't it be fair to characterize the overall aim of psychoanalysis as the attempt to reveal the hidden truth about a human being by uncovering the falsehoods and errors with which she first presents and gives an account of herself to the analyst?[71] The philosophical conundrum of self-deception has even driven some philosophers to formulations that, despite themselves, go more than half way to meet some of the requirements of psychoanalysis, in particular the account of repression and the unconscious.[72] Sartre was neither the first nor the last, though he may have been the most sharp-witted, to see that the language of repression and resistance cannot render redundant the language of lying, of duplicity and doubleness.

> Thus psychoanalysis substitutes for the notion of bad faith, the idea of a lie without a liar; it allows me to understand how it is possible for me to be lied to without lying to myself since it places me in the same relation to myself that the Other is in respect to me; it replaces the duality of the deceiver and the deceived, the essential condition of the lie, by that of the "id" and the "ego." It introduces into my subjectivity the deepest intersubjective structure of the *mit-sein*. Can this explanation satisfy us?[73]

The answer to Sartre's question must be: since any explanation for bad faith, for self-deception, even for weakness of the will, is required to introduce such a structure of subsystems, of intersubjectivity, into the subject, the psychoanalytic explanation does not suffer on this account. We don't know how we do it, but we know that we do: we lie to ourselves, and to that extent, we almost certainly lie to others in exactly the same way. And asking which came first, the lie to the other or the lie to oneself, is probably not only a chicken-and-egg question, but refers only to a mythical chicken and egg.

In fact, in certain respects, lying is a more propitious concept for psychoanalysis than fantasy. The lie already brings with it the theme of transference: it implicates the other in the scene, whereas fantasy could be thought to be purely a reporting of mental contents. In order to introduce the transference into the analysis of fantasy, one insists that there will always be a transferential dimension, whether implicit or explicit, to fantasy, and then insists, in the style of Melanie Klein, that interpretation must always bear upon this transferential aspect of the fantasy. But the way into the transference via lying (and in general via any of the themes where it is the addressee that is in question) obviously opens up immediately the question of the epistemological dimension of the transference. Ferenczi, as so often, pointedly raised this question with the simple title of his briefest of published observations: "To Whom Does One Relate One's Dreams?" The observation consists of two sentences, the first of which is: "We analysts know that one feels impelled to relate one's dreams to the very person to whom the content relates."[74] When Lacan added knowledge to love and hate as the third essential dimension of the transference, he knew full well that knowledge emerges in the relation between analyst and patient primarily in the form of deception and lies.

We thus see—yet again—how the debate over the question of reality or fantasy in the early history of psychoanalysis is misplaced. What Freud did with his shift from the lie to fantasy (thus conferring accreditation on the speech of the hysteric) was to require himself to invent the concept of transference in order to reinstate the reality of the object. The fruitful discarding of the seduction theory, which is linked, I have argued, with Freud's working out of the transferential position of the patient-analyst system, necessitated that psychoanalysis rediscover its reality in the transference. Lying is the negative starting-point which had to be left behind for psychoanalysis to exist, but at the same time psychoanalysis will, to use Lacan's phrase, always operate in the dimension of the lie, because it is always negotiating the dialectic of lying and truth in the speech of an other.[75]

Remember the old lady who as a girl found her independence—one is tempted to say: herself—in the lie that her mother never discovered? The importance of "(not) knowing one's thoughts" was emphasized by Lacan:[76] the discovery that the Other (parent) does not know my thoughts is the moment when the not-said is brought into my being—the moment when one becomes a subject possessing the dimension of the unconscious. The formulation "my parents know my thoughts" is the foundation of speech—all of thought is to be found in the Other (the discourse of the Other). Lacan notes: "then the child realizes that the adult does not know its thoughts—there lies the path of repression." One crucial means of transition from "my parents know my thoughts" to "the Other doesn't know what I am thinking" is the lie; as Lacan writes: "even if it is destined to deceive, the discourse speculates on faith in testimony."[77]

The liar that Christopher Bollas discusses in his book *The Shadow of the Object* used lies precisely to get under his analyst's skin. He told dramatic lies to his analyst and to others, to entertain, confuse, and finally to disappoint and let them down. In one session, he inquired how strictly the analyst was bound to respect the confidentiality of his patient's communications, particularly in relation to the police. The analyst kept his cards close to his chest, attempting to leave himself room for maneuver, by making it clear that he could not give promises about what he would or would not do—as we have seen, it is definitive of the classical position for the analyst never to give promises. In the next session, the patient informed Bollas of the confidence at issue: he was planning to commit a murder.

In the subsequent sessions, the patient went into systematic detail about the plan. The analyst writes: "Over the [next few] weeks I became more anxious, and my interpretations that this was a murder in the transference, and that he was enjoying this presentation had no seeming effect. He politely told me that, if anything, such comments helped him as he felt that I was so out of touch with him that I was an innocent and that, when he had carried out the murder, I could feel that I had not truly known what he was doing, since I had always sincerely thought that it was transference."[78] Under this pressure, the analyst could not sustain the position in which his patient had placed him, that of the "innocent" bystander.

> After a while, I wondered. Possibly he really was planning to kill this person. The more I pondered this situation, the less I knew what to do. I decided to discuss matters with a colleague who, in a helpful and matter of fact sort of way, simply said, "tell him that if he does kill this person, you most certainly will tell the police." She suggested that I would have to decide whether at some point I should inform the potential victim so he could take safety.

Now, as I look back on this episode after the passage of time, it does all seem rather extraordinary. How could I have come to such a point of confusion? In fact I think that in this lie Jonathan conveyed in the transference, and precipitated in the countertransference, the core of the liar's distress: some inability to distinguish between reality and phantasy. It is this psychotic quality concealed in the omnipotence of lying that Jonathan brought into the analysis through my countertransference, for I found I could not distinguish between reality and phantasy.[79]

Prompted by his colleague, Bollas told his patient that he would tell the police if he committed the murder, and that he reserved the right to act as he chose if he thought the murder was actually going to go ahead. This had the effect of clarifying for the analyst that the murder plan was not (never had been? was no longer?) projected into external reality.

Bollas reflects that the liar "elaborates fictions which he chooses to relate as if they were real, and he brings along the other as an unknowing accomplice in the life of the lie"[80]—so unknowing in this instance that the analyst had to bring in his colleague as a third party, a second accomplice. The analyst is required to play to the hilt the role of the unknowing accomplice. And when the truth suddenly bursts in on the lie, the analyst *knows* and *shares* with the patient "the madness of the lie," and shares the shocked feeling of the departure of the fictional reality that he had up until then not known, in a sense, was either fictional or real. The lie and its disappearance transmit the experience of a trauma: the experience of a mediated reality which disappears with no warning.

So Bollas, like O'Shaugnessy, is not experiencing a special sort of crisis in relation to a patient who lies. The meeting of a liar and a psychoanalyst is not the one thing the analyst should dread, like a priest confronted with a happy atheistic sinner. The liar with his murder plan may well be out to murder his friend and his analysis at the same time, but in that respect he does not differ from other patients who repeat their traumas with their analyst, making the latter angry, wretched, hopeless, bereft of feeling or chronically confused. That is what analysts *expect* their patients to do. And patients, one might say, expect their analysts to be there precisely for that. The lie is not the atomic bomb of the analytic war between patient and analyst. It is not the defensive weapon that irreversibly changes the nature of analytic warfare.

There still remains the question: what does the liar use the lie and the lied to for? Bollas argues that the analyst must be the liar's unwitting accomplice. But this answer is too general. It is an answer that flows too easily from the ordinary presuppositions of modern object relations theory, which assume that the analyst will inevitably come to play the part of the patient's principal historical object or objects, and that, insofar as the patient is unconsciously bringing this about, the analyst will only become aware of exactly what object, role, or part he is unwittingly playing through a long, drawn-out, and fundamentally confusing process. The benign analogy for the question: for what does the liar use the lied to? is: what is fiction used for? No doubt the very existence of fiction awakens the desire to transgress the boundary between fantasy and reality. People feel let down by the fictionality of fiction, just as they feel let down ("mad" is the word Bollas insistently uses) when they realize that the other has been consistently lying to them. Thus there are many people who pine over (the non-reality of) Jane Austen's Darcy in the same way as they pine for an old lover, or who mourn Hamlet in much the same way as they mourn John Lennon. But the more general question of the uses of fiction, as of lying, requires an account of under what social conditions fiction is benign, socially beneficial, and of primary cultural importance. In the Western European tradition, we have forgotten these questions, in the way Nietzsche describes how the liar forgets the origin of his truths in metaphor; but we should be reminded of their importance, and maybe even of their fragility, by some cultural crises of recent years. There is the affair of Salman Rushdie's fiction *The Satanic Verses*, which demonstrates to us just how limited the social space of fictionality might become under a different regime of truth. There is the slow recovery of the Eastern European cultures from the Great Lie of the twentieth century. And there is the crisis of memory, fantasy, and truth that pits—in clinics, therapists' offices, police stations, social security offices, and the courts—survivors of abuse against the False Memory Syndrome Foundation.[81]

Nor can it be taken for granted that the space of analysis, akin to that socially sanctioned space of fiction, will remain an uncontested safe haven. Another story of analytic murder, taken from R. D. Laing's autobiographical memoir, illustrates this keenly.

When working as a junior psychiatrist in Glasgow in 1955, Laing had made friends with Karl Abenheimer, a 70-year-old German-Jewish refugee, legally trained and a lay psychotherapist. One night Abenheimer shared with Laing a problem patient, a consultant anes-thetist who "had led him to suppose (had told him directly, in so many words) that he had killed three people in the last year by curtailing their oxygen in the course of long, complex, surgical op-erations. He kept his overall statistics normal, so that he had no more statistically significant anaesthetic deaths than the average for his sort of job. Anyway, he had had a good run for the last three months so was now about to kill the next victim. He would choose someone with a bad heart, poor lungs, or what not, so that their death would not raise any eyebrows."

Abenheimer felt himself required to confront the problem of the lying patient:

Could this chap simply be having him on? Over the years, all psychia-trists are told some extraordinary stories and it is not always easy to know what to believe, even at the best of times. There is a condition called *pseudologia phantastica* in which the patient elaborates fantastic events and yarns, sometimes very plausibly, so that it can be difficult, impossible to be sure . . . Nevertheless, Abenheimer had become al-most sure (how could he be *absolutely* sure?) that his patient was telling the truth. It was fantasy acted out in fact. Now he was asking himself whether he should do anything.

The psychoanalytic imperative would be to continue interpreting, in the hope of getting through to the unconscious sources of the plan. But, after a year of treatment, interpretation did not seem to work: "It did not make any difference. Indeed, the anesthetist had come along to him to get treatment for just this piece of pathological behavior."

> Should Abenheimer tell the patient that what he was doing was *wrong* and risk getting confused with his super-ego? Should he refuse to go on seeing him if he did not promise to stop it? Was not his best chance of stopping it not in fact to stay in existential psychotherapy, the aim of which was to help him to realise why he was fulfilling the compulsion about which he was complaining? Should he approach the superintendent of the hospital he worked in? But he was not medically qualified. His patient might well deny it all and brazen it out, putting him, Abenheimer, in a queer position.
>
> So? What would you do? In *his* position. A German-Jewish naturalized refugee without medical qualifications in Glasgow in 1955, talking to an ex-captain RAMC, a young psychiatrist at Glasgow University?[82]

The first thing to be said about this story, now paired with Bollas's countertransferential psychosis induced by his lying patient, is that we are seeing the dilemma not through the eyes of the first unknowing accomplice, the analyst, but of the second, the colleague who is called upon to offer helpful advice. Laing does not tell what advice he offered, nor does he recount the denouement of the story. As in so many other of his writings, he leaves the reader in the dilemma, the *Zwickmühle*, the double bind. One course of action would betray the analysis, the other course of action would betray the potential victim of the murderer. Laing's narrative, what is more, intensifies the dilemma by reducing the social reality of the psychotherapist—a non-medical German-Jewish refugee in Glasgow—to zero. Such a man, Laing implies, is, as seen from the grim realities of postwar Scotland, himself a fantasy figure, not someone to be taken seriously.

It may also have been possible that the anesthetist was deluding himself about having committed murder. After all, what was the evidence? For a committee that surveyed the evidence of his professional competence, there would be no evidence of wrongdoing: his statistics were in order. From a statistical point of view, no murder had been or would be committed. The utilitarian calculus would find in his "falsehood" no measure of harm done to others. The anesthetist was clearly prey to the fantasy of being rather godlike in his behavior—with one hand he could give life, by keeping his death-count lower than that of other anesthetists, and with the other hand he could take it away by intentionally manipulating the flow of oxygen. He giveth and he taketh away. Perhaps his description of his behavior as murder was equally godlike. Could he, let alone we, be sure that his intention had really been to kill these patients—could it not have been a retrospective interpretation of their deaths as murder, in the service of his self-aggrandizement? After all, every anesthetist is "responsible" for the deaths of patients, in the sense of being the anesthetist in charge when surgical events within their domain of expertise lead to a death. What narratives do all those other anesthetists create in order to give an account of themselves? There will certainly be great variation in such narratives; Abenheimer's anesthetist may have been deluded by the weight of his own responsibility, his desire to play God, and the unexceptional fact of having a regular number of patients die in his care into thinking that he was a murderer. Does such a narrative become pathological simply through giving the narrator the lead part? It might be said that the alarm call, the call on the police or the hospital authorities, would have been tailor-made to fit into and to exacerbate, rather than resolve, the god-delusion of the anesthetist—when in reality a god-delusion is simply the chronic occupational disease of anesthetists, his version of housemaid's knee.

The question also arises whether the anesthetist was a fantasy patient—not in the sense that Laing or his colleague made up the anesthetist, but in the sense that this real anesthetist did not want to be analyzed, but rather wished to be handed over to safer hands, for instance the police. It is, after all, a peculiar demand to make of an analyst: the demand for a cure for his murderous actions which, to judge from the way in which they are reported by Laing, he rather enjoys and does not feel uncomfortable with. There is no hint of pain or conflict in this story, and, insofar as it shares that atmosphere with Bollas's patient's methodical murder plan, one wonders if the analyst had not become, like Bollas, an unknowing accomplice to something other than this murder plan. Perhaps, like Bollas's patient, the anesthetist's aim was to murder his analysis, to put it to sleep permanently. And, as the analyst seeking advice realized only too well, there is no better way of murdering analysis than by being obliged to call in the police or any of those other authorities to which Laing gives the collective name of "super-ego."[83]

Laing's dilemma has been resolved by law in the United States on the precedent of the *Tarasoff* case of 1976. Tatiana Tarasoff was a young woman killed by Prosenjit Poddar in 1969. Poddar had been intermittently under the care and surveillance of psychologists attached to the University of California at Berkeley, and had informed his therapist that he intended to kill Tarasoff. The therapist informed the police, who detained and then released Poddar, but did not inform Tarasoff or her parents. When Poddar carried out his plan, Tarasoff's family took the university to court for negligence. The majority opinion in the case determined that "public policy favoring protection of the confidential character of patient-psychotherapist communications must yield to the extent to which disclosure is essential to avert danger to others. The protective privilege ends where the public peril begins."[84]

In the United States, this duty to warn is now a legal duty for psychotherapists—although, as Beauchamp and Childress rather mordantly observe, "a moral obligation to obey the law is present, but this obligation, like the obligation to confidentiality, is prima facie; and sometimes the health care professional is justified in breaking the law in order to fulfill a responsibility to a patient."[85] That is, the obligation to obey the law is not founded on anything more than the fact that the law is the law; this obligation is a superficial one, whatever the urgency we so often feel about obeying it—it simply inheres in the very idea of law. If there are more compelling, because "deeper," reasons for not obeying the law, then the doctor (or therapist) is morally obliged to ignore the law. While this argument may be cogent, it is now the case in the United States that the rigorous preservation of confidentiality is outside the law, whereas prior to this case it was within it.

The change this ruling brings about in the status of what the patient says to the analyst is captured well by the dissenting opinion in *Tarasoff*:

> The impairment of treatment and risk of improper commitment resulting from the new duty to warn will not be limited to a few patients but will extend to a large number of the mentally ill. Although under existing psychiatric procedures only a relatively few receiving treatment will ever present a risk of violence, the number making threats is huge, and it is the latter group—not just the former—whose treatment will be impaired and whose risk of commitment will be increased.[86]

Justice Clark here underlined the fact that there are a number of groups at risk: (1) those who are the victims of violent crimes committed by those receiving treatment; (2) those who commit violent crimes while receiving treatment; and (3) those—a "huge" number—who make violent threats and do not carry them out. Basing his consequentialist argument on the utility that confidentiality has in the treatment of the mentally ill, he refused to sacrifice the interests of the second and third category, those who threaten violence, to the interests of those who are the victims of violence. It is the hugeness, one suspects, of the number who threaten without carrying out which carried considerable weight with him. Put in other language: those who voice fantasies of violence, who may, like Bollas's patient, construct sophisticated lies centered on murdering someone, should be protected by confidentiality. More to the point, the psychoanalyst should be allowed to maintain a space of freedom in which such threats, fantasies, and lies can be voiced, without automatically triggering a warning system for those who are named as potential victims. However, because of the majority ruling, the psychoanalyst is now legally obliged to transmit such a threat to the potential victim; he or she cannot, within the law, interpret this threat as a lie or a fantasy.

The *Tarasoff* case has broken down the framework of confidentiality upon which the psychoanalyst's suspension of the distinction between lies and truth, fantasy and reality depends. The analyst's ear has become a potentially transparent conduit to the police file and thence to the court of law, where the rules governing the relation between reality and fantasy are entirely different from those in psychoanalysis. As early as 1906, Freud had addressed this issue when talking to a group of legal officers. He had reflected that, by its very nature, psychoanalysis would not offer much aid to the law in the task of ascertaining whether a person was lying or telling the truth, guilty or innocent, since psychoanalysis is not interested in establishing guilt or innocence, reality or fantasy:

> You [legal workers] may be led astray by a neurotic who, although he is innocent, reacts as if he were guilty, because a lurking sense of guilt that already exists in him seizes upon the accusation made in the particular instance. You must not regard this possibility as an idle fiction; you have only to think of life in the nursery, where such events are often enough to be observed. It sometimes happens that a child who has been accused of a misdeed strongly denies the charge but at the same time weeps like a detected sinner. You may perhaps think that the child is lying when he asserts his innocence; but this is not necessarily so . . . Many people are like this, and it is still open to question whether your technique will succeed in distinguishing self-accusing individuals of this kind from those who are really guilty.[87]

Freud was indicating to these legal officials that psychoanalysis pursued its truths down different paths from those of the law and had very good reasons for so doing. What matters in psychoanalysis is the fact that a patient has *said* something, not whether that something is true or not. In the 1970s, it was the turn of the law to inform the psychoanalysts that their pursuit of the truth would from now on always be subject to a legal, rather than psychoanalytic, final court of appeal. The benefit of the doubt would always be on the side of truth, not lies or fantasies.

———

Truth, which only doth judge itself, teacheth that the inquiry of truth, which is the love-making or wooing of it, the knowledge of truth, which is the presence of it, and the belief of truth, which is the enjoying of it, is the sovereign good of human nature.

Francis Bacon, *Of Truth*

We have seen how the absolute prohibition on lying of the moralist philosophers can be countered in a number of different ways— through a naturalistic defense, through a utilitarian defense, through an anthropology of society and the individual imagination. We have seen how science and medicine negotiate between truth and lies in the human domain while still attempting to maintain an ideal of objective scientific truth. And we have seen that the novelty of the solution of psychoanalysis to the threat of lying and deception resides in its transcending of the dialectic of belief and deception. But there is a pervasive, almost involuntary shock and withdrawal at the prospect either of being deceived or of being a deceiver—among moralists, social scientists, and even among those analysts committed to transference analysis and the unfolding of the subject's relations to its (imaginary) objects. Must psychoanalysts necessarily react to the liar with shock and the impulse to withdraw? Is this reaction inevitable for a profession that believes, as Carol Gilligan aptly characterizes the common starting point of feminism and psychoanalysis, that it is lies that make you ill and truth that cures you?[88] Is that yearning for the far side of lies—in other words, a nostalgia for the truth—constitutive of psychoanalysis, no matter how much equanimity and technical poise analysts bring to the mixture of fictions and truth that is necessarily their daily fare?

It is the Enlightenment Freud, the scientific Freud, the ethical Freud, call him what you will, who is attached to the belief in the truth. The other Freud, the psychoanalyst in action, behaves otherwise. He mobilizes the questioning, the healthy questioning, that we find in Nietzsche's short essay on science, piety, and truth: "This unconditional will to truth—what is it? Is it the will *not to allow oneself to be deceived?* Or is it the will *not to deceive?* . . . But why not deceive? But why not allow oneself to be deceived?"[89]

Nietzsche pushes us to ask why we might be so attached to the truth, to not being deceived, to not deceiving—to this complex of ideals which constitutes the "piety" on which science is based. If we believe in the value of truth because it is prudent and useful to do so, because of the utility of science, what should we do when lying, deception, and cunning prove their own mettle, when Homer, the first individual, holds up for us the moral of the great deceiver Odysseus? Such reminders of the uses of deception will carry weight even before we turn to notice how much is destroyed and sacrificed in the name of truth. We thus have to look for a moral basis for science and the value of truth which is prior to and independent of the good or evil that truth does in the world. "*Why have morality at all* when life, nature, and history are 'not moral'? No doubt, those who are truthful in that audacious and ultimate sense that is presupposed by faith in science *thus affirm another world* than the world of life, nature, and history; and insofar as they affirm this 'other world'—look, must they not by the same token negate its counterpart, this world, *our* world?"[90] This audacious and ultimate truth may therefore be on the side of the eternal as opposed to the ever-changing world of lies and appearances. It may be on the side of death as opposed to life. Yet this truth, insofar as it does not belong to our world, may be precisely the lie by which we, the children of science, now live.

# GIFT, MONEY, AND DEBT

> Therefore the proud man can afford to wait, because he has no
> doubt of the strength of his capital, and can also live, by anticipa-
> tion, on that fame which he has persuaded himself that he deserves.
> He often draws indeed too largely upon posterity, but even here he
> is safe; for should the bills be dishonoured, this cannot happen until
> *that debt* which cancels all others, shall have been paid.
>
> Charles Colton, *Lacon* (1822)

> *mngwotngwotiki:* The Tangu of New Guinea's description of para-
> dise, meaning a particular field of relations in which the individuals
> concerned are temporarily unobliged to each other.
>
> K. Burridge, *New Heaven, New Earth*

For someone who advocated a return to Freud, Lacan was little prone
to quoting him. "Quoting," he is quoted as saying—though I can't
exactly remember when and where—"is for imbeciles." So, if we find
the name "Freud" in Lacan's work, it is very rarely followed by the
words invoked by Marie Bonaparte so frequently that they became
her nickname: "Freud-a-dit." In this respect—and I am only stating
the obvious—Lacan quoted Freud far less often than other psychoanalysts do and did, and certainly far less often than, say, Lacanians
cite Lacan.[1]

So the famous return to Freud is *not* a return to the letter, if only
because what is commonly regarded as the letter of Freud, the text
itself, is largely missing from Lacan's work. The return thus can only
have been, and palpably was, to the spirit of Freud. And Lacan's own
practice implied that those who return to the letter of the text are
imbeciles, if that is where they think they will discover its spirit.

Yet Lacan exhorted others to return to Freud, meaning return to those very texts he himself eschewed citing. To take an example, from the last page of "La chose freudienne" ("The Freudian Thing"):

> One has only to turn the pages of his works for it to become abundantly clear that Freud regarded a study of languages and institutions, of the resonances, whether attested or not in memory, of literature and of the significations involved in works of art as necessary to an understanding of the text of our experience . . . Indeed, Freud himself is a striking instance of his own belief: he derived his inspiration, his ways of thinking and his technical weapons from just such a study.[2]

Even if you flick through Freud's pages, not bothering to read, you will see that Lacan's reading of Freud is correct. This is quite typical of one important mode of citation in Lacan's work.

The implication is: anyone can understand what Freud is saying, since it is written down in black and white, in plain German, French, or English for all to see; and yet, it is also implied, no one before Lacan has managed to do this simple thing. For example, he writes in "The Freudian Thing": "Freud's intention, which is so legible to anyone who is not content simply to stumble through his text . . ."[3] So it is somewhat surprising to discover that the most extended piece of analysis and commentary of any text of Freud's to be found in Lacan's *Ecrits* is in an appendix: "Commentaire parlé sur la *Verneinung* de Freud." The author is Jean Hyppolite.

So Lacan's reading of Freud is always something different from commentary, from the traditional art of *explication de textes*. To speculate somewhat: the diffidence and reluctance Lacan betrayed in relation to the telling of case histories may be of the same sort, have the same source, as his reluctance to quote Freud. And, we should remember, this reluctance to confront the text of the experience of reading Freud when discussing it with others, this reluctance to confront the text of his analyses when discussing the technique of analysis with others, is a distinctive feature of the theorist who proposed the transmission of the experience of analysis to others in "la passe" (the passage or the pass) as one of the fundamental tasks for the analyst. Speculatively, then, we surmise that this analyst, whose textual indirection was so prominent a part of his relation to his colleagues and students, also felt the pressure to find some theory of how textual directness was possible—of how the experience of analysis, or of reading Freud, could be transmitted to others.

However, this is not entirely true or just. One knows that Lacan did succeed both in transmitting his own experience of reading Freud to others and in giving a clear sense of analytic practice as he conceived and executed it. How did he do this, being so firmly committed to indirection?

According to Lacan, the fundamental prerequisite for reading Freud is the principle of faith: one must place one's faith in Freud's writing, otherwise one won't know where to start. In one of the main texts to be discussed in this essay, "Le mythe individuel du névrosé, ou 'Poésie et Vérité' dans la névrose" ("The Individual Myth of the Neurotic, or 'Poetry and Truth' [*Dichtung und Wahrheit*] in Neurosis"),[4] Lacan recognizes that all of Freud's case histories are "incomplete," that they seem to many analysts to be "analyses broken off midway," and that they are only "fragments of analysis." But this, he goes on, "must all the same stimulate us to reflect, to ask ourselves why the author has made this choice, *and of course to place our trust in Freud.*"[5]

This register of *trust*—of faith not only in the other's good intentions but in his intelligence—precedes and organizes any reading of Freud which will be able to do justice to his work. In other words, in order to read Freud, one must place Freud in one's debt *before the reading starts.* One must give Freud the benefit of the doubt—and extend this seemingly temporary charitable act indefinitely.

"Trust," "have faith": this register is not only the register of the necessary cement of social life in general, not only the register of a nonrational relation to God, it is also the register of financial exchange. When Lacan refers to symbolic exchange, or to symbolic debt, we must not neglect to inquire into the structure of this economic system—to the point where I would suggest that the principles which govern the Symbolic system might well be called an "economics of the symbol."

So, in order to read Freud, one must postulate that he has, in effect, issued a currency, a psychoanalytic currency, and that in holding the text, we are holding the notes of credit of this economic system. Placing trust in Freud is thus like placing trust in the institution that issues notes of credit or banknotes. Freud's texts thus must be treated as promissory notes, if one is going to be able to read them properly.

We often catch such overtones in Lacan's conception of the relationship between Freud and his readers: as we have seen, his reader is anyone who can read, anyone who can turn a page. Indeed, Lacan sometimes places himself in a role where the only reason he is willing to speak is in order to help other potential readers of Freud free themselves of what is blinding them, of what is preventing them from reading Freud: "I would take this opportunity of reminding those who cannot be persuaded to seek in Freud's texts an extension of the enlightenment that their pedagogues dispense to them . . ."[6]

Lacan's "reminder" is only necessary, is perhaps only *defensible*, he implies, because it is obliged to function as a substitute, a *semblant* (counterpart), of Freud's texts. It is as if some readers, some analysts, treat Freud's texts as in need of something additional, something that, when it accompanies the text, makes it trustworthy, a proper currency. In Britain, people who have bank accounts are issued pieces of plastic called check guarantee cards, intended to supplement the guarantee offered by their signature. Lacan is, in effect, implying that readers and analysts treat Freud's texts as if they were checks issued by any private citizen, and therefore in need of a check guarantee card. If only they could recognize, through placing the appropriate trust in Freud's texts, that these are not like checks, but are instead the equivalent of banknotes issued by the National Bank, then they would give up requiring supplementary guarantees from others (such as Lacan), in the same way that nobody requires a respected National Bank to issue a guarantee card with each banknote. The note is its own guarantee; one need look no further. Freud's text is its own guarantee; one need look no further.

However, having placed such trust in the text, Lacan then points out one fundamental condition of this trust. Freud's case histories are trustworthy precisely to the extent that they are free of doctrinal constriction, to the point where they appear to the trained psycho-analytic eye as contrary to the basic technical rules of psychoanalysis: "The successes obtained by Freud, because of the heedlessness about matters of doctrine from which they seem to proceed, are now a matter of astonishment, and the display so evident in the cases of Dora, the Rat Man, and the Wolf Man seems to us to be little short of scandalous."[7] These texts are trustworthy precisely because they are, each and every one, unique deviants. They do not obey their own rules. And therefore they can still be used to correct them, to reach down to the fundamental doctrines they embody and sink new doctrinal foundations for them to rest upon. In Lacan's 1953 lecture "The Neurotic's Individual Myth," he used the case of the Rat Man to show the limitations of the Oedipal schema precisely with Freud's own clinical evidence. Freud's case history is shown to be a resource that embodies its own curtailment and correction. This necessary deviation from Freud's own text is sanctioned by the refusal of slavish imitation. Lacan is the last person who would explicitly recommend being a slave to another master: "It is not a question of imitating him. In order to rediscover the effect of Freud's speech, it is not to its terms that we shall recourse, but to the principles that govern it."[8]

It is also not clear the extent to which Lacan viewed Freud as a sleepwalker, that is, whether he made his discoveries, acted in accordance with these principles, despite himself or in full and deliberate knowledge. It is certain that now, after Freud's death, when psycho-analytic doctrine has taken over from these principles, in order to recover those principles one cannot repeat these texts. Lacan's discourse of the Freudian golden age, forever lost to us moderns, entails that we can only recover the essence of that age by reinventing it in an alternative mythical guise. So Lacan will not quote; he will not follow Freud; he will give something much simpler and yet more subtle: he gives us an account, a *compte rendu.*

Lacan's gifts as a storyteller have not been widely advertised. As quasi-epigrammatist, as spinner of semantic spider's webs, as tortuous and complex edifier of theories, he is well known. But Lacan as simple storyteller? Yet he opens his *Ecrits* with a seminar on a story, and much of the exhilarating novelty of his reading of Poe's story is embedded in a retelling of the tale. He was immensely gifted in this art of retelling, and with each of Freud's case histories, as well as Poe's story, Sophocles' *Antigone,* not to mention the case histories he selects and dissects from the psychoanalytic literature, he retells the story in such a way that the Lacanian point is embedded in the process of recounting. This is a gift.

Thus Lacan had the gift of making his *compte rendu* of Freud's cases or papers in the form of a story. In this way he paid off the debt he owed to Freud for this material. "The Neurotic's Individual Myth" is also the theory of the debt which is enacted in the reading. Its ethos is tragic; the debt is *impayable:* there is no settling of accounts possible—not, at least, in this life—without death. To clarify the concept of debt, I want to consider Lacan's various readings of Freud's case history of the Rat Man.

———

The young patient who became known as the Rat Man came to Freud in 1907. Freud's treatment of him lasted several months, and he found him a congenial and apt example of a classical, moderate obsessional neurosis. The patient acquired his name from the frightening story of a rat torture that he had heard from a captain while he was doing his military service, a torture which he felt compelled to imagine was being performed on his fiancée and his father—despite the latter having been dead for some time. The immediate cause of his coming to Freud was a bewilderingly complex set of tasks and duties he had set himself in connection with a pair of spectacles that had been sent to him from Vienna, via the Post Office, while he was on maneuvers. But Freud found the heart of his obsessional thinking to lie in a conflict over whether or not to marry his fiancée, a conflict that resonated with the path his father had taken in life and was prompted in part by his mother's plans for his future.

Lacan's discussions of the case focus on two main themes, the first a doctrinal element, the second a question of analytic technique. The doctrine is that of *debt*. The technical point arises out of a consideration of Freud's errors. The consideration of the doctrine and the technique, which are intimately linked together, will clarify both the concept of debt and its enactment in Lacan's relation to Freud.

In his case notes on a session some two months into the treatment, Freud recorded: "I pointed out to him that this attempt to deny the reality of his father's death is the basis of his whole neurosis."[9] This interpretation that Freud offered the Rat Man after two months of treatment was not available to Lacan when he gave his 1953 lecture, yet it sums up very well the heart of Lacan's reading of Freud's published case history. If the Rat Man is attempting to deny the reality of his father's death, this explains why he is pursued by his father in his imagination. That is, he is pursued by an imaginary father. To begin with, we should recognize how Lacan's reading of Freud's text isolates the precipitating cause as the original scene of the analysis, and links it closely with its repetition, the scene of the payment of the debt—the *délire* of the repayment of the 3.80 kronen the Rat Man owes to someone for the safe delivery of his pince-nez.

The organization of the account is very similar to that more famous *compte-rendu*, "Seminar on *The Purloined Letter*." In Lacan's analysis of *The Purloined Letter*, what structurally organizes the two scenes, and also provides continuity between them, is the letter. In the *compte rendu* of the Rat Man, it is a debt that organizes the two separate scenes, making the recent scenes the repetition of the two others, the scene of the Rat Man's father's premarital indebtedness and the scene of his marriage. In *The Purloined Letter* there is the triangle of the King, Queen, and Minister repeated with the characters of the police, the Minister, and Dupin. For the Rat Man, however, there is no one simple scene that is repeated once; rather we find two primary scenes that are then each repeated.

The first scene is that of the patient's father's debt to the mysterious friend, which is then repeated with Lieutenant A., the lady at the post office, and Lieutenant B. The second scene is that of the Rat Man's father and two women: the rich and the poor girl. This scene of the father and the rich/poor girls is repeated with his son, in the debt repayment drama involving the lady at the post office and the innkeeper's daughter, and also in the structure that precipitated the neurosis in the first place: the scene of the Rat Man, the cousin whom it is proposed he should marry, and his lady. Lacan characteristically sums this up:

> You cannot fail to recognize in this scenario—which includes the passing of a certain sum of money from Lieutenant A. to the generous lady at the post office who met the payment, then from the lady to another masculine figure—a schema which, complementary in certain points and supplementary in others, parallel in one way and inverted in another, is the equivalent of the original situation.[10]

According to Freud, and following him Lacan, the Rat Man's neurosis began when his mother told him of her plan for him to follow in his dead father's footsteps and marry a young, rich, and beautiful member of her family.

> This family plan stirred up in him a conflict as to whether he should remain faithful to the lady he loved in spite of her poverty, or whether he should follow in his father's footsteps and marry the lovely, rich and well-connected girl who had been assigned to him. And he resolved this conflict, which was in fact one between his love and the persisting influence of his father's wishes, by falling ill; or, to put it more correctly, by falling ill he avoided the task of resolving it in real life.[11]

His father had at one point also confronted the choice with which the Rat Man's mother was now presenting her son: the choice between marrying a rich or a poor girl. In his father's case, the poor girl had been a butcher's daughter[12] and the rich girl was the Rat Man's mother, who brought with her, for the uneducated father, the security of the family business.

Lacan follows Freud's account closely in seeing this family "constellation" as being the pathogenic cause of the patient's neurosis. He also follows Freud in seeing that it had become pathogenic through its being a repetition of the father's own early experiences—through its being what Freud, in his case notes, called "his regression to the story of his father's marriage."[13] But, whereas Freud refers crucial elements of this story to "chance," adding that "chance may play a part in the formation of a symptom, just as the wording may help in the making of a joke,"[14] Lacan makes these specific chance elements effects of a structure whose existence he will put forward as being more fundamental than the explanation Freud offers, in terms of the conflict between the father's prohibition and the son's libidinal desire. The two chance elements of Freud's that are focused on are, first, the debt, and, second, the choice between the rich and the "poor, but pretty" girls.

His father, in his capacity as non-commissioned officer, had control over a small sum of money and had on one occasion lost it at cards. (Thus he had been a *"Spielratte."*) He would have found himself in a serious position if one of his comrades had not advanced him the amount. After he had left the army and become well-off, he had tried to find this friend in need so as to pay him back the money, but had not managed to trace him. The patient was uncertain whether he had ever succeeded in returning the money. The recollection of this sin of his father's youth was painful to him, for, in spite of appearances, his unconscious was filled with hostile strictures upon his father's character. The captain's words, "You must pay back the 3.80 *kronen* to Lieutenant A.," had sounded to his ears like an allusion to this unpaid debt of his father's.[15]

Lacan places greater emphasis than Freud on this friend, and high-lights—by forgetting to mention it earlier—the fact that the debt was never repaid: "On the one hand, we have originally the father's debt to the friend; I failed to mention that he never found the friend again (this is what remains mysterious in the original story) and that he never succeeded in repaying his debt."[16] Lacan displays his acute "intuition" here, since Freud himself had, in his unpublished case notes, focused on exactly this same question, in an urgent note to himself:

He lost some of it in a game of cards with some other men, let himself be tempted to go on playing and lost the whole of it. He lamented to one of his companions that he would have to shoot himself. "By all means shoot yourself," said the other, "a man who does a thing like this ought to shoot himself," but then lent him the money. After ending his military service, his father tried to find the man, but failed. (Did he ever pay him back?)[17]

It is almost as if Freud made this note as a kick to himself, first for failing to ask his patient the question, and second as a reminder to himself to find out in the next sessions. Lacan, uncannily, having noticed the mystery of the disappearing friend in Freud's published text (not in the case notes), underlines that having noticed it and its importance, he forgot to mention it. This, it seems to me, is proof, if it were needed, of Lacan's acute sensitivity to Freud's way of working—so acute, it seems, that he knew how to forget exactly where Freud forgot, without knowing it.

Yet in a recapitulatory account of this incident, Lacan introduces a new note, that of the mysterious stranger, "the mysterious friend who is never found and who plays such an essential role in the family legend"[18]—one almost sees the black coat, the shadowy profile. Such Hoffmannesque tones would certainly not be out of keeping with Freud's focus, given the decisive advice to commit suicide which the Rat Man's father had received from this stranger-friend—and yet this passage concerning the suicide was again unavailable to Lacan, because it is only to be found in the case notes. So Lacan's tracking of the original moment of the debt to this gambling debt of the Rat Man's father's youth is entirely in keeping with the way in which Freud himself had sewn the Oedipus complex into the lining of the Rat Man's family romance.

Freud and Lacan both agree, then, that the military maneuvers of the Rat Man, with the loss of the pince-nez and the compulsion to pay 3.80 kronen to Lieutenant A., is a repetition of the primal scene of the Rat Man's father's gambling debt, in which he was saved from dishonor, prison, and worse by a mysterious friend, to whom he remained for the rest of his life in debt. The question of the debt is also present in the other primal scene that is repeated: his choice between the poor but pretty girl (the son's poor lady taking over the role of the father's butcher's daughter) and the rich heiress who brings with her professional security. In marrying the Rat Man's mother, the father was placing himself in debt to her—"status comes from the mother's side,"[19] Lacan notes.

Yet Lacan intends to place the accent elsewhere. Instead of underlining the conflict between the father's wishes and the patient's love for his lady, Lacan highlights the narcissistic rivalry with the father and the consequent dissolution and splitting of an object relationship. In this sense, Lacan makes the mysterious creditor-friend a structural feature of the "parental imago." The general principle Lacan invokes is the following: "In this very special form of narcissistic splitting lies the drama of the neurotic."[20] To back up this point, Lacan gives an account of the three terms of each scene whereby the male subject has a doubled, either/or relation to the figures of the idealized woman and the debased woman, and the woman has an equivalent relation to the alienated subject and the social representative, the friend. The splitting of the function of the male subject has as its correlative the complementary splitting of the function of the female object. Lacan insists that these are two variants of one structure; it is this conviction that underpins his rejection of the triangular Oedipal structure in favor of a quaternary structure, which is thus a duplication of a duplication, a doubling of a double. This is the account Lacan gives of the articulation of the different characters in terms of the debt:

> In order to understand thoroughly, one must see that in the original situation, as I described it to you, there is a double debt. There is, on the one hand, the frustration, indeed a kind of castration of the father. On the other hand, there is the never resolved social debt implied in the relationship to the figure of the friend in the background. We have here something quite different from the triangular relation considered to be the typical source of neurotic development. The situation presents a kind of ambiguity, of diplopia—the element of the debt is placed on two levels at once, and it is precisely in the light of the impossibility of bringing these two levels together that the drama of the neurotic is played out. By trying to make one coincide with the other, he makes a perennially unsatisfying turning manoeuvre and never succeeds in closing the loop.[21]

Yet in a text from the same year of 1953, Lacan began to repudiate, or at least question, the element of castration in this account of the Rat Man's debt in favor of a concentration on the notion of the "social debt." The means by which he achieves this is striking, since it involves accusing Freud's text of claiming something that it is difficult to find in that text.

> Freud even goes so far as to take liberties with factual accuracy when it is a question of attaining to the truth of the subject. At one moment he perceives the determining role played by the proposal of marriage brought to the subject by his mother at the origin of the present phase of his neurosis. In any case, as I have shown in my seminar, Freud had had a lightning intuition of it as a result of personal experience. Nevertheless, he does not hesitate to interpret its effect to the subject as that of his dead father's prohibition against his liaison with the lady of his thoughts.
>
> This interpretation is not only factually inaccurate. It is also psychologically inaccurate, for the castrating action of the father, which Freud affirms here with an insistence that might be considered sys-

tematic, played only a secondary role in this case. But the apperception of the dialectical relationship is so apt that Freud's act of interpretation at that moment sets off the decisive lifting of the death-bearing symbols that bind the subject narcissistically both to his dead father and to the idealized lady.[22]

As I have already pointed out, Freud had claimed that it was a conflict between the "persistence of his father's wishes" and the Rat Man's love for his lady that led to his neurosis. This "persistence" is not necessarily, not even primarily, restricted to a prohibition. But it is also clear that Freud did seek to discover the source of the Rat Man's fears about his father's death, and that he interpreted these fears, and the obsessional defenses against them, as evidence of *wishes* for that death.

> At this I told him I thought he had now produced the answer we were waiting for . . . The source from which hostility to his father derived its indestructibility was evidently something in the nature of *sensual desires*, and in that connection he must have felt his father as in some way or other an *interference*.[23]

But, in accusing him of factual inaccuracy, Lacan is imputing to Freud something beyond this insistence that the patient's fear of his dead father stems from early memories of interference with sensual desires. Clearly Lacan is perturbed by the fact that it is the mother's, not the father's, plan that constitutes the implicit prohibition on his marrying his lady. Lacan states that Freud sees the father's speech as prohibiting the marriage with his poor lady love:

> The turning-point came when Freud understood the resentment provoked in the subject by the calculation his mother suggested to him concerning his choice of a spouse. That Freud links the fact that such advice implied for the subject the interdiction of his engagement to the woman he loved to certain words of his father, when this linkage is in conflict with the basic facts of the matter, notably the prize fact

of all that his father is dead, does surprise one, but it is justified in terms of a deeper truth, which he appears to have come upon within himself and which is revealed by the chain of associations which the subject then adds. Its justification is to be found in nothing other than what we call here the "chain of speech," which, while making itself heard in the neurosis and in the fate of the subject, extends well beyond the individual: namely that a similar lack of faith had presided over his father's marriage, and that this ambiguity itself conceals an abuse of trust in a money matter which, in driving his father out of the army, decided his marriage . . .

But if Freud's interpretation, so as to untie this chain, with all its latent significance, will end up dissolving the imaginary web of the neurosis, that is because, in terms of the symbolic debt which is promulgated by the subject's tribunal, this chain renders him comparable less to his legatee than to his living witness.[24]

Some clarification may help here. Lacan conflates the father's opposition to the poor girl with the mother's promotion of the rich girl. One might think that they amount to the same thing, as if the father's opposition to the one will drive him into the arms of the other. But to prohibit and to promote are very different speech acts. Now Freud observed that the Rat Man does experience this conflation between the maternal and the paternal voices: from the patient's point of view, the choice "rich girl versus poor girl" lines up his own desires against those of his family's, in particular against the disapproval the father expresses of the lady ("his father, shortly before his death, had directly opposed what later became our patient's dominating passion. He had noticed that his son was always in the lady's company, and had advised him to keep away from her, saying that it was imprudent of him and that he would make a fool of himself").[25] Yet at no point in his *compte rendu* does Freud impute to the father an *active* prohibition of the marriage to the poor lady. Lacan is, we might say, textually incorrect, but, one must immediately add, true to the entire thrust of Freud's reconstruction—because behind the mother's plan to marry her son into her family and its business is, for the Rat Man, the coincidence of this plan with the choice his father made, marrying (his mother) for money, not love. The Rat Man's conflict concerning his father is not so much over the prohibition as over the identification that is being required of him. And, we might say, the careful term "persistent influence of his father's wishes [*fortwickenden Willen des Vaters*]" which Freud used, interpreted too readily by Lacan as "prohibition," covers both cases.

The same strange insistence occurs when Lacan addresses another of Freud's "errors" in the conduct of the case. In the second session of the treatment, the patient was about to recount the story told him by the cruel captain of the rat torture. Freud writes:

> Here the patient broke off, got up from the sofa, and begged me to spare him the recital of the details. I assured him that I myself had no taste for cruelty, and certainly had no desire to torment him, but that naturally I could not grant him something which was beyond my power. He might just as well ask me to give him the moon. The overcoming of resistances was a law of the treatment, and on no consideration could it be dispensed with . . . I went on to say that I would do all I could, nevertheless, to guess the full meaning of any hints he gave me. Was he perhaps thinking of impailment?—'No, not that; . . .' etc.[26]

Lacan comments that, by these interventions, Freud appears to be taken in by the subject's game. He seems to fall in with the patient's demand that, so that he can continue, he must be given something like a pledge. But no, Lacan says, what Freud offers the patient is not a transgression of some supposed neutrality of the analyst. What Freud offers the patient is "the symbolic gift of speech, replete with a secret pact, in the context of the imaginary participation which includes it, and whose implication will be revealed much later in the symbolic equivalence that the subject fixes in aligning his thoughts of the rats with the florins with which he recompenses the analyst."[27] Once again, what appears to be analytic confusion or wavering on Freud's part turns out to be his sure sense of the primal significance of the interrelations between speech, debt, and the patient's rat economy. At every turn, these are the themes that Lacan will draw out of Freud's case history.

The background to Lacan's flurry of imputed factual inaccuracies and textual imprecisions is the long-term strategy of his reading of the Rat Man, a strategy that will lead to two fundamental revisions of the Freudian account. The first is the need "to make certain structural modifications in the oedipal myth, inasmuch as it is at the heart of the analytic experience."[28] This modification will require Lacan to introduce the concept of the moral master—the Absolute Master, we might say, the antecedent of the concepts of the Other and the Master in Lacan's later writings. In Freud's case history, he argues, we perceive the "fundamental conflict which, through the mediation of rivalry with the father, binds the subject to an essential symbolic value."[29] This binding occurs in relation to an actual debasement of the figure of the father; analysis takes place in the space, the gap, or the ambiguity between the debased and this other figure of the father:

> The analyst nevertheless assumes almost surreptitiously, in the symbolic relationship with the subject, the position of this figure dimmed in the course of history, that of the master—the moral master, the master who initiates the one still in ignorance into the dimension of fundamental human relationships and who opens for him what one might call the way to moral consciousness, even to wisdom, in assuming the human condition.[30]

Whereas in Derrida's reading of *The Purloined Letter*, it is Lacan who is accused of an unwarranted superposition of the triangular Oedipal scenario onto the scene of the theft of the letter (Minister, King, Queen—where is the observer/narrator of this scene? Derrida asks), in the case history of the Rat Man it is Lacan who, in effect, accuses Freud of superimposing an Oedipal triangle (prohibiting father, object mother, desiring subject). The discovery that there are four, not three, elements involved in the neurotic's individual myth requires a revision of the founding myth of psychoanalysis:

> The quaternary system so fundamental to the impasses, the insolubilities in the life situation of neurotics, has a structure quite different from the one traditionally given—the incestuous desire for the mother, the father's prohibition, its obstructive effects, and, around all that, the more or less luxuriant proliferation of symptoms. I think that this difference ought to lead us to question the general anthropology derived from analytic doctrine as it has been taught up to the present. In short, the whole oedipal schema needs to be re-examined.[31]

The splitting of one of the three figures in the Oedipus myth is what requires this revision, and Lacan gives, as I have already noted, an account of how each of the three terms of the Oedipal triangle may be split: the subject (social subject and alienated witness), the object-woman (rich versus poor, legitimate versus passionate object) and the mediating third term, the father (debased, symbolic). However, the scene of splitting, although itself prone to being duplicated in a variety of ways, stems from a single fundamental moment, the specular moment of narcissism, imbued with aggressivity and idealization—and this is the second of Lacan's fundamental revisions of the Freudian account: "The narcissistic relation to a fellow being is the fundamental experience in the development of the imaginary sphere in human beings."[32]

Yet this discovery of the fundamental character of narcissism, usually summed up in accounts of Lacan's work under the rubric of the mirror-phase, was, we now begin to see, closely linked with the question of the position of the father in the symptomatology, the mythology of the neurotic. More than any other analyst, more even than Freud, I suggest, Lacan was concerned with the destiny of the father. The question of the father emerges in an anthropological, even culturalist register in Lacan's writings of the 1930s, already juxtaposed with, contrasted with, and correcting the myth of the primal father found in Freud's *Totem and Taboo:* "Our experience leads us to discern the principal determinant [of the major contemporary neurosis] in the father's personality, which is always lacking in some respect: absent, humiliated, divided against himself or a sham."[33] On the basis of this phenomenology of the neuroses, Lacan suggested an explanation for the very existence of psychoanalysis:

> A great number of psychological phenomena appear to stem from the decline in society of the paternal imago . . . Perhaps the very emergence of psychoanalysis should be linked to this crisis. The sublime chance of genius does not, perhaps, by itself explain that it was in Vienna—then the centre of a State which was the melting pot[34] of extremely diverse familial forms, from the most primitive to the most sophisticated, from the last agnatic groupings of Slav peasants to the most simplified petit-bourgeois households and the most decadent of unstable family menages, by way of feudal and mercantile paternalisms—that a son of the Jewish patriarchy came up with the Oedipus complex.[35]

In this culturalist account of the origins of psychoanalysis, Freud's discovery of the Oedipus complex is linked to his prior investigation of the anomie whose two principal causes are the incomplete repression of desire for the mother, and the "narcissistic degeneration of the idealisation of the father, which highlights, in the Oedipal identification, the aggressive ambivalence immanent in the primitive relation to one's counterpart."[36] At the center of the Oedipus complex, for Lacan in 1938, stands "the father, in so far as he represents authority and in so far as he is the centre of sexual revelation; we have linked to the inherent ambiguity of his imago, the incarnation of repression and catalyst of an essential access to reality, the twofold development, typical of our culture, of a certain character of the super-ego and a particularly evolutive orientation of the personality."[37]

We should not forget that the 1930s was a period when the attention of most psychoanalysts was turning more to the mother and away from the father. Lacan's early work accurately reflects these

127

researches, in particular those of Melanie Klein, and the importance of what he called the "separation complex," which embraced what other analysts would have called anal and oral sexualities. Yet, however modified and central the figure of the mother became, Lacan was insistent on the pivotal role played by the father—even in 1949, when he spoke in the culturalist dialect of the absent, wounded, or unemployed father:

> The maternal imago is far more castrating than the paternal imago. At the end of each of my analyses, I have seen appear the fantasy of dismembering, the myth of Osiris. It is when the father is lacking in some way (dead, absent, blind even), that the most severe neuroses develop.[38]

Lacan's reflections expressed a nostalgia for a society where complex familial structures will, "at each stage in life, become enriched by a growing complexity of hierarchical relations."[39] The themes continued into the 1960s, when he described the obligation of the small boy confronted with the symbolic burden of the phallus as the continuation of "Daddy's rules, and as everyone knows, for some time now Daddy hasn't had any rules at all, and that's where all the problems start."[40] On many occasions, Lacan returns to this grandiose figure of the father whose decline we have participated in, indeed inherited. And he is not always cast in the tragic mode that is in keeping both with Freud's vision of the murdered father at the beginnings of history, and with Lacan's invocation of the "stone guest who comes, in symptoms, to disturb the banquet of one's desires";[41] he is frequently invoked in the comic mode of Count Almaviva, condemned to be forgiven by his spouse instead of exercising his *droit*, or *dette, de seigneur.*

———

Thus, by the 1930s, continuing to the early 1950s, Lacan had established a doctrinal foundation in his assertion of the decline of the father imago and its relation to imaginary narcissistic rivalry. He made it clear that the Oedipus complex was itself a culturally relative structure, linked to the familial and marital structures of modern society, and to the decline of the father. With his examination of the Rat Man case history, he found in the very symptom the patient presented the term which would allow him to take one more step toward elaborating the system of the Symbolic, Imaginary, and Real, with which he would be able to replace, or at least to reinterpret, the Oedipus complex. That term was "debt." As the clear doctrinal exposition of the "discours de Rome" put it:

> The paternal function concentrates in itself both imaginary and real relations, always more or less inadequate to the symbolic relation that essentially constitutes it. It is in the *name of the father* that we must recognize the support of the symbolic function which, from the dawn of history, has identified his person with the figure of the law. This conception enables us to distinguish clearly, in the analysis of a case, the unconscious effects of this function from the narcissistic relations . . .
>
> Thus it is the virtue of the Word that perpetuates the movement of the Great Debt whose economy Rabelais, in a famous metaphor, extended to the stars themselves.[42]

The English translator of the *Ecrits* helpfully provides the reference from Rabelais. Debts, says Panurge, are "the connecting link between Earth and Heaven, the unique mainstay of the human race; one, I believe, without which all mankind would speedily perish." Debts, he continues, are "the great soul of the universe."

Such a passage confirms for us how Lacan conceives of his androcentric psychoanalytic revision: one will not be able to understand or intervene effectively in the Oedipus complex if one does not recognize the "interference" of narcissistic rivalry and fascination which one finds in the figure of the imaginary father; the surest way to secure this recognition is to remain aware of the fundamental symbolic function of the father. As the Rabelais reference indicates, the universe that the symbolic father inhabits is the universe of the Great Debt.

Let us remind ourselves that for the Rat Man, the debt in question was purely imaginary. By the time he came to Freud, the real debt had, thanks to his sensible friend, already been paid off. What was left of his *délire* were occasional impulses to find Lieutenant A. and pay the debt. And these impulses were molded in the direction of finding the doctor who would help him pay off his debt:

> His determination to consult a doctor was woven into his delirium in the following ingenious manner. He thought he would get a doctor to give him a certificate to the effect that it was necessary for him, in order to recover his health, to perform some such action as he had planned in connection with Lieutenant A.; and the lieutenant would no doubt let himself be persuaded by the certificate into accepting the 3.80 crowns from him. The chance that one of my books happened to fall into his hands at that moment directed his choice to me. There was no question of getting a certificate from me, however [*Bei mir war aber von jenem Zeugnis nicht die Rede*], all that he asked of me was, very reasonably, to be freed of his obsessions.[43]

Freud is quite certain that he will not help this deluded patient to pay off any debt whatsoever. Freud will offer him freedom; he will not help him pay his debt.

Yet this debt will, for Lacan, become something magnificent, the emblem of individual destiny, and the signifier of the social order itself. The importance of the debt makes it highly significant that Lacan overlooked this passage in Freud's case history; indeed, in one of his accounts of the case, he distorted his account of the chronology of the case history so that Freud emerges as the friend who *did* help the Rat Man pay his debt: "once the treatment is begun, he is content quite simply [*tout bonnement*] to send a money order to the lady at the post office."[44] Lacan concertinas the chronology here: the Rat Man had paid the generous lady at the post office well before coming to analysis with Freud. Through this discounting of the time that elapsed before the Rat Man met Freud, Lacan elides the presence of the sensible friend. He in effect coalesces the helpful assistance of the sensible friend with what Freud had to offer his patient, making it seem as if Freud had something to do with the payment of the debt to the lady at the post office:

> His friend had held up his hands in amazement to think that he could still be in doubt whether he was suffering from an obsession, and had calmed him down for the night, so that he had slept excellently. Next morning they had gone together to the post office, to dispatch the 3.80 *kronen* to the post office at which the packet containing the pince-nez had arrived.[45]

In this elision, we glimpse the long-term strategy of Lacan's revision of psychoanalytic theory. Through his reading of the Rat Man case history, he will install the notion of debt as a crucial element of the quaternary structure that replaces the Oedipus complex. This debt is no longer imaginary; it will be called "symbolic debt." It is the phrase *tout bonnement* ("quite simply") that is revealing: as if starting the treatment with Freud, in his analytic role the quintessence of the symbolic function, was sufficient to release the patient from his incapacity to pay off his debt. And the fact that Lacan puts Freud in place of the friend shows how Lacan will shift the Rat Man's debt from the register of the imaginary to that of the symbolic.

This elision of the friend and the analyst in the course of the line of interpretation which leads to the centrality of the symbolic debt is associated with another curious amalgamation we find in Lacan's commentaries on this case: the rapprochement of the analyst and the patient. On two different occasions, with respect to two different elements, Lacan amalgamates the unconscious of the analyst and that of the patient.

The first of these concerns Freud's own arranged marriage. Lacan points out on two occasions that Freud was able to perceive the determining role of the mother's marriage plan in the Rat Man's neurosis as a result of a personal experience.[46] On the second of these occasions, in "Variantes de la cure-type" ("Variants of the Typical Cure"), he specifies what incident he is referring to:

> Now it appears that Freud's gaining access to the crucial point of the meaning, in which the subject can literally decipher his destiny, was made possible by the fact of having himself been the object of a similar suggestion stemming from prudential family considerations—which we know about through a portion of his self-analysis to be found in his writings, unmasked by Bernfeld—and if, on that occasion, he hadn't responded with opposition, that might have been enough for him to have missed the moment, in the treatment, of recognizing it.[47]

Lacan is here alluding to the paper "Screen Memories," in which Freud demonstrated how his earliest memory, of playing in the field near Freiburg with his two playmates John and Pauline, was a product of the repression of two later events: his calf-love for Gisela Fluss at the age of sixteen, and his father's and brother's plan to marry him and Pauline, his cousin, and settle them in Manchester.[48] Lacan is surmising that in order to be able to recognize the determining effect of the Rat Man's mother's proposed marriage on the neurosis, Freud himself must earlier have reacted, when he was nineteen, with opposition to the plan his family had cooked up; if he had not, if he had acquiesced in the plan, he would not have been able to recognize this incident as the cause of the neurosis. This is a strong claim, despite its being couched in characteristically oblique fashion. It proposes, in effect, that the neurotic formation of Freud's that corresponds to the Rat Man's obsessional neurosis was his screen-memory, and that it was through the similarity of structure of these two neurotic formations that Freud was able to isolate the precipitating cause, the fundamental determinant, of the recent phase of the Rat Man's neurosis. What Lacan does not point out, which he might have done, is that Freud had already *analyzed* this particular neurotic symptom, his screen-memory, and therefore benefited by some knowledge of the structure that was organized around the marriage proposal, as opposed to having been in a position to identify, or undergo an involuntary identification, with the unconscious structure in his patient.

In the spirit of Lacan's hypothesis, we might also add another element which brought Freud's and the Rat Man's personal experiences together: the analysis of Freud's own dream of *Company at table or table d'hôte*, which centered on the idea of what has to be paid for love, and the debts we necessarily incur in our friendships and family relations.[49] The desire was expressed in the dream through the theme of "beautiful eyes." Freud's crowning interpretation was that he wished to be loved for his *beaux yeux* only, he wished for love that was not *countable*, not rendered into the register of gratitude and debt—love beyond the debt principle. So when, in a murky period of work with the Rat Man, the patient had a dream of seeing Freud's daughter with two patches of dung instead of eyes, Freud applied the interpretation that had worked for him to his patient: "should he remain faithful to the lady he loved in spite of her poverty, or should he follow in his father's footsteps?" Should he marry for love or for money? Should he step outside the circle of paternal debt or honor it? However, where Freud's dream registered a protest against love always having to be paid for, the Rat Man's dream, with the alacrity born of its ironic intention, eagerly forced love into the framework of a marriage with Freud's daughter which was for her money, not her beauty. Whereas Freud, the forty-four-year-old father of six, already inhabited the register of marriage, yet regretted the curtailments that that implied, the young, single Rat Man refused to recognize the register itself, except in his dreams and symptoms, since marriage meant for him the identification with his (dead) father and the renunciation of love in favor of money (rats).

Such rapprochements between Freud and his patient are plausible. But the second of Lacan's rapprochements is far more curious, because it is so obscure and almost undetectable—if it is in any sense detectable. It occurs in the rhetorically baroque and obscure penultimate section of Lacan's 1955 paper "The Freudian Thing," the section entitled "La dette symbolique" ("Symbolic Debt"). The title indicates that, for my reading of Lacan's reading of Freud, this is a key passage:

> Will our action go as far, then, as to repress the very truth that it bears in its exercise? Will it send this truth back to sleep, a truth that Freud in the passion of the Rat Man would maintain presented for ever to our recognition, even if we must increasingly divert our vigilance away from it: namely, that it is out of the forfeits and vain oaths, lapses in speech and unconsidered words, the constellation of which presided at the putting into the world of a man, that is moulded the stone guest who comes, in symptoms, to disturb the banquet of one's desires?
>
> For the unripe grape of speech by which the child receives too early from a father the authentification of the nothingness of existence, and the bunch of wrath that replies to the words of this false hope with which the mother has baited him in feeding him with the milk of her true despair, set his teeth on edge more than having been weaned on/from an imaginary *jouissance* or even having been deprived of such real attentions.[50]

The mention of the Rat Man's passion leads one to believe that the two allusions that follow are to *his* experience; far from it. The two references of the second paragraph are, I infer, taken not from the Rat Man's childhood, but from Freud's own catalogue of childhood experiences. The first refers to the judgment passed by his father on the son who had urinated in his parents' bedroom: "the boy will come to nothing"—a judgment which pursued Freud in his dreams for the rest of his life, obliging him to enumerate constantly for his imaginary father the substantiality of his existence.[51]

There is, it is true, an episode in the Rat Man's childhood which has some similarities with Freud's memory: when the father declares that his son's elemental fury indicates he will be either a great man or a great criminal.[52] Freud adds in a note, as if wanting to confirm the importance of such prophecies, that the father overlooked the most likely outcome of such premature passions: a neurosis. But this incident from the Rat Man's childhood could not be, despite the obliquity of Lacan's prose, what is referred to with the phrase "the authentification of the nothingness of existence"; at most, it provided Lacan with a switchword to the Freudian allusion.

The second allusion, to the mother's despair, is, I suspect—beyond the evocation of the powerful final scene of Steinbeck's *The Grapes of Wrath*, where a famished young man is nourished at the breast of a young woman whose baby has died—to the vivid demonstration of human mortality that Freud's mother once gave him:

> When I was six years old and was given my first lessons by my mother, I was expected to believe that we were all made of earth and must therefore return to earth. This did not suit me and I expressed doubts of the doctrine. My mother thereupon rubbed the palms of her hands together—just as she did in making dumplings, except that there was no dough between them—and showed me the blackish scales of *epidermis* produced by the friction as a proof that we were made of earth.[53]

And, Freud continues, "I acquiesced in the belief which I was later to hear expressed in the words: *'du bist der Natur einen Tod schuldig'*—'thou owest Nature a death.'"[54] With this tracing of implicit associations, we have, I think, arrived at Lacan's *terminus ad quem*.

With this passage, we have stumbled upon the strangest, most allusive subtext to Lacan's commentary on the Rat Man: passing by way of an elision between the Rat Man's and Freud's childhood experiences, we come upon the unpayable debt of each speaking being, which Lacan, in less Shakespearean, less directly religious mode, will call, a page later, "the symbolic debt for which the subject as subject of speech is responsible."[55] Passing from the Rat Man, through a circuitous reading of Freud, we arrive at the final doctrinal end-point: the symbolic debt of the subject insofar as he is speaking, the debt he owes to the Other.

———

Debt as a fundamental property of the Symbolic is the mature Lacanian axiom. The notion of symbolic debt is indissolubly linked to the notion of the symbolic father, whose genesis from the 1930s on we have followed:

> The attribution of procreation to the father can only be the effect of a pure signifier, of a recognition, not of a real father, but of what religion has taught us to refer to as the Name-of-the-Father.
>
> Of course, there is no need of a signifier to be a father, any more than to be dead, but without a signifier, no one would ever know anything about either state of being.
>
> I would take this opportunity of reminding those who cannot be persuaded to seek in Freud's texts an extension of the enlightenment that their pedagogues dispense to them how insistently Freud stresses the affinity of the two signifying relations that I have just referred to, whenever the neurotic subject (especially the obsessional) manifests this affinity through the conjunction of the themes of the father and death.
>
> How, indeed, could Freud fail to recognize such an affinity, when the necessity of his reflexion led him to link the appearance of the signifier of the Father, as author of the Law, with death, even to the murder of the Father—thus showing that if this murder is the fruitful moment of debt through which the subject binds himself for life to the Law, the symbolic Father is, in so far as he signifies this Law, the dead Father.[56]

The debt is now Lacan's manner of purifying the notion of guilt and of morality of its "instinctual" sources. The ambiguity of the Rat Man's debt—the imaginary debt to the friend as separate from the symbolic debt to his father, which can only be recognized once he ceases, as Freud put it, denying the death of his father—is now the means by which Lacan can articulate the junction of the symbolic and the imaginary. And with the register of debt, Lacan can fuse the notion of exchange, borrowed from the anthropology of Marcel Mauss *(The Gift)* and Claude Lévi-Strauss, with the exchange of words, the pure symbols that constitute the articulation of the Symbolic, and, most intriguingly, with the register of money. For can we forget that among the most common uses of the polysemic debt are those linked to money and the system of finance? Certainly neither the Rat Man nor Freud forgot it: the first response of the patient to being told the financial arrangements involved in psychoanalysis was to think to himself: "So many florins, so many rats!" And it was surely as much on account of the curious currency he brought to the analysis as for his memorable rat torture that Freud gave the patient his sobriquet.

There is one striking passage in Lacan's writings where he draws the analogy, not infrequent elsewhere, between money and speech. The context of the passage, written in 1953 in the Rome Discours, is Lacan's denunciations of present-day psychoanalytic technique: the specific target is the mixing up of the registers of the Imaginary and the Symbolic that too close an attention to the dimension of the here and now can entail. The danger is the analyst's promotion, once again, of the alienation of the subject in an objectification of his ego, his imaginary point of identification. What the analyst must do, rather, is deprive the subject's certainties of support. Suddenly, Lacan evokes a deserted discourse:

> However empty, in fact, may appear this discourse, all one can do is take it at face value: that justified by Mallarmé's sentence in which he compares the common usage of language to the exchange of a coinage whose sides now only reveal effaced figures, a coinage passed from hand to hand "in silence." This metaphor is sufficient to remind us that speech, even when it has, through everyday wear and tear, reached its limit, retains its function as token.
>
> Even if it communicates nothing, discourse represents the existence of communication; even if it denies the evidence, it affirms that speech constitutes truth; even if it is destined to deceive, it speculates on faith in witnessing.[57]

The contrast evoked by the image of the effaced coin being passed from hand to hand in silence is one between the melodramas of popular psychoanalysis—stories of grandiose identifications, horrific stories of past abuse, tempestuous bouts of transference-passion—

and a stark vision of humans deprived of all that is colorful, historical, meaningful. On the beach, stranded in a world we know from
Beckett and Bergman, humans wordlessly measure out their beings-
for-Death by exchanging an effaced coin, a subway token that still
functions as a token even after the Bomb has fallen.

In *Seminar I*, Lacan used the same metaphor to illustrate talking
to no purpose. While he obviously had Heidegger's rather coarse
category of "idle talk" in mind, the image from Mallarmé is, nonetheless, a subversion of the Heideggerian put-down of idle talk.
Lacan emphasizes how talking to no purpose (how could one do such
a thing?—that is exactly how Freud defines free association, so that
unconscious purposive ideas now come to the fore) reveals one of the
fundamental truths of language:

> But even [talking to no purpose], as I've explained elsewhere, has its
> meaning. This realisation of language, now only serving *as an effaced
> coin passed from hand to hand in silence*—a phrase I quoted in my Rome
> report, which comes from Mallarmé—indicates the pure function of
> language, which is to assure us that we are, and nothing more. That
> one is capable of speaking to no purpose is just as significant as the
> fact that, when one speaks, in general it is for a purpose.[58]

The passage from Mallarmé to which Lacan is referring is the
following: "to relate, to teach, even to describe is fine and although
perhaps enough for each individual to exchange human thought, by
taking or putting a coin silently in someone else's hand, the elementary use of talk serves the universal *reportage* in which, with the
exception of literature, everything among the different kinds of
contemporary writing partakes."[59] There is, we see, a significant
difference between Mallarmé's image and Lacan's version of it. For
Mallarmé, everyday life is simply sustained by the taking and receiving, in silence, of little coins, as if the essential structures of communications were given in the small gestures of touching and the
little kisses of welcome and goodbye rather than the twittering of
tongues that fills up the rest of life spent "In Company." Lacan adds

the trope of the effaced figure to Mallarmé. He adds, thereby, the dimension of a past, a past present in the signs of its having been annulled. Lacan's additional figure means that we live, not in the flat two-dimensional reality of Mallarmé's everyday life without past or future, but in the twilight zone of effaced coins, canceled meanings, historical monuments.

Strangely enough, Lacan could have found a term that uses the figure on a coin as the guiding figure of speech to describe the patient's discourse in Freud's very first case history in *Studies on Hysteria*, Frau Cäcilie M. or Baroness Anna von Lieben, who suffered from a "hysterical psychosis for the payment of old debts."[60] All the old debts had been accumulated, Freud had indicated, by her making false connections in the past: her neurotic symptoms were masks, excessive stories, covering over the true and hidden connections, which her cathartic cure would reveal. Getting the true words out, expressing them adequately, in the proper place, to the proper person: this is another way of describing her either paying off or writing off these old debts. The speech emitted can almost be counted off, on one side of the balance sheet, against the debt, the past obligations, represented, as if they were old IOUs, by symptoms.

The German word that Freud used to describe his patient is a wonderfully rich and ambiguous term: *hysterische Tilgungspsychose*. *Tilgung* means the deletion sign in typography; *tilgen* means "to extinguish," "to strike out," "to wipe out, to efface," "to delete" (in typography); *Schuld tilgen* means "to pay, compound, discharge, cancel"; *Anleihe tilgen* means "to redeem," and thus *Tilgungschein* means "certificate of redemption." Anna von Lieben spent much labor redeeming all her old debts, issuing certificates of redemption through the hard work of catharsis she accomplished with Freud. It took her three years of the talking cure, Freud writes, to redeem the old debts of thirty-three years.

There is little doubt that in these very early writings, Freud on occasion allowed the three registers of confession, moral sin, and financial debt to intermingle, a play made easy by the resonances of

the term *Schuld* in German. The cathartic cure is a confession of
sins, and it is also a *Rechnung,* a reckoning, a toting up of the sins of
the past, sometimes even the sins of the father that have been visited
upon the daughters and sons. There is an equivalence between the
speech of the patient, on the one hand, and the old debts that are
being brought to account and finally paid off, on the other.

We are not, quite, speaking of money and speech here; but the
register is not far from it. The register is that of obligation. We could
coalesce them, it seems, by making a distinction between responsible
and irresponsible speech. The speech of psychoanalysis appears to
be speech at its most irresponsible: free association, whose relevance
or social acceptability is intentionally placed to one side. The injunction is an odd one: do not take responsibility for your speech! In this
way, you will discover that you are far more responsible for it than
you ever realized or imagined. One starts off, as Lacan put it, in the
exactly opposite direction to your intended goal: you start off mouth-
ing nonsense, only to discover these are precious truths. You start
with oaths and blasphemy, only to discover these are sacred words.

So Lacan could have looked back, as he so often had done, to Freud
for the interweaving of monetary terms with the register of obligation
and responsibility. But he would have found only a faint echo of the
image of the effaced, annulled, *tilgt* coin in Freud. Where else do we
find this figure of the effaced coin? In Nietzsche: "So what is truth?
. . . truths are illusions we have forgotten are illusions; they are
metaphors which have become habitual and drained of sensory force,
coins which have been effaced and which from then on are taken to
be, not pieces of money, but metal."[61] Truth, Nietzsche asserts, is the
passing of the effaced metal coin of metaphor from one hand to
another. Metaphor falls to the level of truth through the effacing of
the figure emblazoned on it; truth is the effacing of metaphor. It is
the effacing that allows people not to recognize what has taken place,
so that they can forget and rely on the comfort of truth.

The figure of effacement introduces, for both Nietzsche and Lacan, a two-phase history: the "now" of the passage of coin from hand

to hand, which follows the "then" of full recognition of the stamp of the coin: its value, its provenance, which monarch or state issued it, under what circumstances, and so forth. For Lacan, the effacement of the coins resonates with his own theory of the imaginary: the theory of the mirror phase. One can see this clearly in the very terms he employs: "une monnaie dont l'avers comme l'envers ne montrent plus que des figures effacées" ("a coin whose obverse like its inverse now only reveals effaced figures"). To use the terms *avers* and *envers* for the two sides of a coin is, one might say, rather *pervers*. It does, one must admit, communicate clearly the stubborn indeterminacy of the Lacanian subject confronted with the mirror: which is the real image?

But a further reading of Lacan's insertion of the effaced figure shows that it follows through the distinction he was in the process of making in this passage, between full and empty speech. Full speech would be, then, the exchange of coins whose figures have not been effaced, the original inscriptions whose loss is recorded in hysterical symptoms.[62] In *Seminar I*, drawing upon his customary linguistic sensitivity, Lacan lends Freud a term borrowed from the more recent work of Lorenz and Tinbergen in ethology, the term *Prägung*, translated into English as "imprinting," but which has the connotation of the striking of a coin. This is the term, Lacan asserts, that best characterizes primal repression, when a traumatic impression forces its way upon the subject.[63] One side of the coin of the word *Prägung* leans toward the imprinting of a figure, and it captures as well the moment of the sudden appearance that is also a crystallization—the process that is usually characterized by the term *Fixierung*, fixation, with all its overtones derived from the sequence of processes by which a photographic image is produced in the darkroom. The chief difference is that the temporality of the two processes run in opposite directions. In a darkroom, one develops and then fixes the image produced; in the Freudian darkroom, the image is fixed but invisible until it is developed by the mechanism of deferred action, *Nachträglichkeit*. Nietzsche's image has the same temporal structure as Freud's: the coin is first struck, corresponding to primal repression, but only becomes truth, becomes metal rather than currency, becomes visible through secondary repression and symptom formation, when the figure is effaced. Full speech is the restoring of the figure to the coin, the restoring of the original metaphoricity of the illusion created by the word.

The more orthodox interpretation of full speech also, as I will now try to show, brings us back to an analogy with money. A number of commentators, among them Shoshana Felman,[64] Jean Bellemin-Noël,[65] Mikkel Borch-Jacobsen,[66] and myself,[67] have pointed out the similarity between Lacan's notion of full speech, or founding speech, and Austin's theories of performatives. For Lacan and Austin, the exemplary performatives, the acts of full speech, are ritual acts of naming, of binding one person to another in a permanent and irreversible bond: "you are my master," "you are my wife." Austin stays closer to the ritual wording: "I do" in the marriage ceremony, "I name this ship" in a launching, and "IOU" in affirmations of indebtedness. The clearest example of the performative is the promise, the core of any contract, whether in its marital or monetary ritual observances. Consider the words on the English banknote—"I promise to pay the bearer on demand the sum of £5." This is the pure performative, a speech act which is its own guarantee, a pure commitment to the other and to the common future of subject and other.

The words "I promise to pay the bearer" correspond to the effaced figure on the coin. Part of the power of the image of the silent passing on of effaced coins derives from the solidity of the coin as a piece of metal, as if we would still treasure the coin once all the other people had silently departed, leaving us alone with no further reason for parting with it. This image of the circulating coin still has the power to revive the conviction that the metal of the coin is something valuable in and of itself, as if it were gold. With a banknote, the dimension of value is evoked more effectively through negativity, through our recognition that the worthless piece of paper is closer to the primary function of money—that it can be exchanged for something other than itself. Lacan's image of the silent passing on of coins emphasizes the structure of exchange, at the cost of the heterogeneity implicit in the idea of an exchange economy: one object is exchanged for another, a *different* object. The promise of money is that one neutral object can give the holder of the banknote or the coin access to an indefinitely large number of other objects, corresponding to the indefinite variety of his or her desires. Empty speech, Lacan implies, remains restricted to exchanging one object for another, identical object. The silent image of money changing hands is equivalent to an affirmation of the act of promising, but with no specification of what is promised—as if one silently pressed into someone else's hand a scrap of paper with no design, no images of a sovereign, simply bearing the words "I promise."

However, I make use of the example of the banknote primarily for reasons beyond its clarity and expository simplicity. More immediately than the coin, the banknote evokes the register of debt. As we have seen, the Lacanian subject becomes a subject only in incurring a symbolic debt to the father, or to the element in the world which instantiates the paternal metaphor. The metaphor is sustained and expanded so as to include the elementary structures of all social relations, through the transplanting of Lévi-Strauss's famous hypothesis that it is the act of exchange of women by men that constitutes the fundamental cement of all societies.[68] Lacan clarifies this hypothesis by giving equal weight to the concept of a debt circulating in the opposite direction to that of the women. As a man exchanges one woman for another, he becomes a symbolic father (one only becomes a father by giving up the imaginary phallus). The woman he receives in exchange brings with her the surplus value of the child. This child's relation to the father is that of indebtedness: the positivity (the actuality) of the male child's material existence is repeated on the level of symbolic existence in the negativity of his debt, which he can only pay off by giving away a woman. This model, drawn from the so-called elementary societies, is itself indebted to Mauss's essay on the gift. Mauss, Lévi-Strauss, and Lacan all agree that the basic social fact is the stable, equilibrated system of symbolic exchanges of gifts. Lacan's rhetoric captures the assumption well:

> Identified with the sacred *hau* or with the omnipresent *mana*, the inviolable Debt is the guarantee that the voyage on which wives and goods are embarked will bring back to their point of departure in a never-failing cycle other women and other goods, all carrying an identical entity: what Lévi-Strauss calls a "zero-symbol," thus reducing the power of Speech to the form of an algebraic sign.[69]

The anthropologists' vision of the stable circulation of all goods, women, and symbols sparks off Lacan's most rapturously deterministic evocation of the force of destiny—what he will later call the combinatory of the Symbolic.

We must now ask: Is Lacan's theory of the Symbolic then one in which a theory of money and of debt coincides with the anthropological theory of exchange? Lacan certainly takes it as axiomatic that the act of giving entails obligation on the part of the recipient. Money, in this theory, is simply the objective measure of obligation, the measure of debt. Certain features of this theory can then be transferred to any exchangeable item. Lacan's axiom is that the Symbolic is grounded on the gift of one specific human property, that of speech: "it is by way of this gift [of speech] that all reality has come to man and it is by his continued act that he maintains it."[70] Hence all other symbolic elements can be, and are, exchanged via the universal medium of speech; speech itself is both medium and element transmitted. Thus, for instance, the function of symbolic love can be deduced from the theory of potlatch in Mauss: love is the gift of what one hasn't, just as one accumulates debts to the destroyers of pigs through being present at the potlatch feast in which the objects of symbolic exchange—"pots made to remain empty, shields

144

too heavy to be carried, sheaves of wheat that wither, lances stuck into the ground"[71]—are "the signifiers of the pact that they constitute as signified."[72]

―――――――

I sense that this grand metaphor of the circulation of symbols between subjects, kinship groups, and entire civilizations has been insufficiently examined. The most seductive aspect of this theory is not the grand union between economics, kinship, the contract theory of society, and linguistics. It is the metaphor which is perhaps most familiar to us in economics, both practical and theoretical, but which has a far wider, older, and deeper hold: it is the metaphor of circulation itself. Within the natural sciences, circular motion was to Aristotle the motion of the perfect, unchanging extraterrestrial world. The Keplerian and Newtonian reforms, followed by the rational mechanics of the eighteenth century, did away with the privilege of the circle and the distinction between the heavens and earth, but installed a new version of this ideal: the equation with determinate solutions and reversible time parameters. Despite the fact that the term given to the political transformations at the end of the eighteenth century was derived from the same geometric and circular ideal—"revolution", after all, refers to the revolving of the spheres— these transformations, together with the parallel transformations of the technology of production known as the Industrial Revolution, introduced the possibility of the world being dominated by processes that are not fundamentally those of the equilibrium of the balance and mathematical recurrence.

The key response to this possibility was the device of the Carnot cycle—the uncanny return of Aristotle's metaphysics as a thought experiment, the founding moment of thermodynamics. Imagine a system which goes through a determinate number of processes which lead it back to its starting-point. This is the description of the ideal system, the ideal heat engine for Carnot. The Carnot cycle made possible one of the most fundamental of scientific innovations of the nineteenth century: the division of all processes into reversible and irreversible ones. The impossibility of perpetual motion—the impossibility of there being such a thing as a wheel that revolves forever and produces useful work, otherwise known as the second law of thermodynamics—ensured that nature is the domain of irreversible processes, whereas the domain of science (of the ideal, the mathematical) is first and foremost that of the reversible—the ideal of circulation still ruling as an ideal type. Even within mathematical physics, paradoxes worthy of the Greeks were produced by this return of the circular: Zermelo's paradox utilizing Poincaré's recurrence theorem, which proved that, in stark contradiction of the second law of thermodynamics, any mechanical system will eventually return arbitrarily close to its starting-point.[73]

When the scientistic worldview of nineteenth-century thermodynamics was evoked to criticize Freud's hydraulic metaphors and old-fashioned science—by those claiming themselves as humanistic psychoanalysts—it was this model of the circulating, lawlike balance-sheet of energy that was at issue. Lacan's defense of Freud saw to the heart of the question: he defended Freud's hydraulics of the libido on the grounds that Freud was simply invoking a material-like substance to give body to what was more properly a network of equivalences, relations of quasi-mathematical equality. This act—giving money to a servant-girl—stands in for two other acts—defecating and copulating. The ecological sensibility, historically akin to political economy and to the balance-sheets of energy and chemical ingredients of agricultural economies, would also express such equivalences, and could provoke such grand projects (with their intendant anxieties) as the recycling of the sewage of the new English industrial towns in order to restore to the countryside the vital elements it was in danger of losing. The cycle of nature's basic currency and the circulation of goods and money could be mapped onto one another.[74]

In the twentieth century the scientism, if such it was, of the balance-sheet of energy transformations, of chemical transformations, and of the human body as a chemical engine could be replaced by the equivalence that was posited between energy and information, culminating in Brillouin's concept of negentropy.[75] The nineteenth-century metaphysics of the balance-sheet of energy and its shadowy nemesis, entropy, could be easily mapped onto the twentieth-century chart of the transmission of information in networks without loss. If Carnot's cycle provided the exemplar for the metaphysics of reversible cycles, it is the electrical circuit and then the computer circuit that have provided the technological devices, the phenomenotechnical realizations, to use Bachelard's term, for our everyday embedding and disembedding in this metaphysics of the circular and the circulation.[76]

The idea of the closed system, linked to but also independent of these developments associated with thermodynamics, can also be found in biological thought, when we trace the genealogy of the idea of the homeostatic system (Cannon and even Breuer) back to Bichat and Bernard, and forward to its development by Wiener and others in cybernetics. With cybernetics, the links between biology and thermodynamics become clear, as do the connections with developments in logic and engineering giving rise to information theory. Cybernetics offers the ideal of a pure science of the system grounded on the model of the collection of elements that always return to the same place, indicating how the circular ideal is realized in nature.

Lacan was acutely sensitive to this novel approach; his deft and astute eclecticism allowed him to combine the burgeoning structuralism of Lévi-Strauss and others with the cybernetic revolution of Wiener, Grey Walter, and their colleagues. Each of these scientific developments, though, represents the recurrence of the scientific ideal of the circular—of the return to the starting-point, and the ordering of every element of a system in relation to this fundamental ideal, which, according to the second law of thermodynamics, can never be more than temporarily real. Hence Lacan's definition of the Real: those things are real which are always in the same place.[77]

One could, of course, reinterpret this history in the opposite sense: one could argue that the history of modern science is the battle against the ideal of the circle and the eternal return of the same. First, Aristotle's *physis* is denatured of circles. The Industrial Revolution and thermodynamics recognize the ubiquity of irreversibility and the ontological status of time—of time's arrow—in the very conceptual development that allows a powerful description of cyclical reversible processes. The project then becomes the description of open and closed systems and the conditions under which they do or do not obey the logic of circular return. Conceiving of organisms, then of societies, then of machines in such terms is a series of attempts to bring to self-consciousness and under analytical scrutiny the ideal of circularity. But the ideal of the system—self-equilibrating, self-correcting, wiping out its history as if it were a Carnot cycle in full operation in the real of society, of language, of ecology—nonetheless dominates even while it is the object of skeptical criticism and regulation. And our technology of circuits insistently reminds us that we associate the circle with life and we associate its dissolution, dispersion, and dismembering with the line going dead. It is this recurrently seductive metaphysics of the circle that reemerges in Lacan's theory of debt.

Another way of putting this is to say: it is the unique, the anomalous, the excessive, the gratuitous, the superfluous that is continually being excluded from the logic of the circular. The clearest statement of this insight can be found in Derrida's brilliant essay *Given Time,* which is addressed to the concept of the gift, especially in Mauss's classic statement. The Maussian theory of the gift is of an economy ordered by the logic of reciprocity and exchange that is included in the act of giving, in prestation (Mauss's term, meaning, roughly, "that which is rendered to the other"). Yet there is another concept of the gift, just as fundamental as that of required reciprocity, as pure gratuity—the tip that is always beyond the price that has been agreed upon by the contracting parties, the excess that is beyond calculation. Wherever the gift as pure gift in this sense exists—if it can exist—it destroys the logic of the gift in the other sense, in the sense of a countable logic of reciprocity and exchange. The gift both requires an answer and annuls any possibility of an answer. The gift is pure act that sets in train nothing other than itself—if it does so, the sense of spontaneity and surplus beyond what is required by the preexisting obligations is annulled. The gift that requires reciprocation annuls itself as gift in that very requirement. The Christmas present that demands the thank-you letter annuls the pure gift of the gift, by pretending that the letter is not itself part of the system of exchanges that make up and, in the very act of letter writing and sending, create ever new sets of exchanges and obligations.

Is such a thing as the gift possible? This is Derrida's unanswerable question. "The truth of the gift . . . suffices to annul the gift. The truth of the gift is equivalent to the non-gift or to the non-truth of the gift. This proposition obviously defies common sense. That is why it is caught in the impossible of a very singular double-bind, the bond without bond of a bind and a non-bind. On the one hand, Mauss reminds us that there is no gift without bond, without bind, without obligation or ligature; but on the other hand, there is no gift that does not have to untie itself from obligation, from debt, contract, exchange, and thus from the bind."[78] The gift will always remain logically impossible, then, though there may be such a thing that, in its lightning appearance, suspends that impossibility—is another name for that impossibility.

> One cannot deny the *phenomenon*, nor that which presents this precisely phenomenal aspect of exchanged gifts. But the apparent, visible contradiction of these two values—gift and exchange—must be problematized. What must be interrogated, it seems, is precisely this being-together, the at-the-same-time, the synthesis, the symmetry, the syntax, or the system, the *syn* that joins together two processes that are by rights as incompatible as that of the gift and that of exchange.[79]

Derrida puts his thesis at its most clear-cut as follows:

> To reduce [the gift] to exchange is quite simply to annul the very possibility of the gift. This annulment is perhaps inevitable or fatal.

No doubt its possibility must always remain open. Still one has to deal
with this annulment, still one has to render an account of the law of
its possibility or its process, of what happens or can not happen in the
form of the gift, to the gift and by way of the gift.[80]

Derrida uses the term "exchangist," linked to "linguisticist and structuralist," to characterize the strategy of Lévi-Strauss, following and
criticizing Mauss, a strategy that is crucial to the paradigm or
episteme of French structuralism of the 1960s.[81] What is this strategy,
which Lacan shared—in part, and the extent to which he participated
and diverged will concern us later—with Lévi-Strauss and the others?

The strategy is to set aside Mauss's residues of magical thinking
which stem from his being too closely identified with or attentive to
specific terms—such as *hau*, which designates both buying and selling, lending and borrowing, giving and taking—to seek beneath the
surface of social reality the iron law of circulation and exchange that
regulates the ethnographic or psychoanalytic unconscious. Lévi-
Strauss perceived Mauss as having been bewitched and proposed the
concept of the zero-symbol in order to designate the concept of
exchange that Mauss had adopted wholesale from the indigenous
conception of the Maoris. Anything can come to occupy this position,
he argues, so it is an empty signifier, a zero signifier. Yet in so doing,
Lévi-Strauss undoes the entire drift of Mauss's argument in *The Gift*,
which was concerned to *distinguish* economies founded on gifts from
those founded upon money, economies ("theirs") founded upon exchange (equivalent to the creation of social bonds) from those
("ours") in which exchange annihilates all bonds except those embodied in the circulation of money.

Thus Mauss locates in *hau* what is necessarily absent in money.
Lévi-Strauss, and Lacan following him, replaces the gift economy
with the signifier economy. In so doing, they eradicate the distinction
Mauss sought to make. All social relations—read the Symbolic—are
to be understood in terms of the peregrinations of the zero signifier,

just as Marx and Simmel's analyses of the modern world demonstrate how the internal logic of money is inherently universalistic, necessarily devouring all sources of value other than money as pure exchange-value. So the linguistic reading of the Maussian political economy, which shifts the emphasis from the universal law of the gift to the universal law of the signifier, undoes the very distinction Mauss intended to make between gift and money economies, and, in so doing, requires us to identify money and the theory of the zero-signifier.

To put this another way: If we read all economies as systems of exchange, in which we cannot usefully distinguish economies that are bonded through the circulation of pigs, of *hau*, or of money, but must subsume them all under the single category of the exchange and circulation of symbols, then the speech act of promising and the coins and banknotes founded on that promise give us the founding act of all human societies. Lévi-Strauss recognizes this at times, seeing in the idea of the social contract "the most profound and most generalizable—that is, verifiable over a large number of societies— idea of what political organization can be, and even the theoretical conditions of any possible political organization."[82] The eighteenth-century foundations of the social contract, also invoked implicitly by Austin, Lacan, and Searle, are the foundations of speech acts in general: good faith, trust, and confidence.

The key notion becomes circulation, rather than reciprocity and exchange. As long as something circulates, or better, in Derridean dialect, as long as *there is circulation*, the second logic of the gift—the exchangist, the linguisticist, the structuralist, the economicist—appears to prevail over the first logic—of the gratuity, of creativity, of charity, of the givingness of giving. Mauss's essay certainly pushes in this direction, seemingly oblivious to the way in which his relentless anatomy of the *hau*, the potlatch, the *kula*—which he translates as "circle or ring, a regular movement in time and space"[83]—erodes the very distinction it is meant to provide, that between social exchange and monetary exchange. Lacan and Lévi-Strauss demolish this distinction by locating the *hau* in the zero-signifier of language, a signifier defined only by its negativity, its difference from all other signifiers. But the other register, which Lévi-Strauss will call the affective or magical register in Mauss, will also return. Let us anatomize this return—this failure of the model of circulation.

———————

The sense that something is missing in a total system of exchange and circulation is clearly present in our intuitions about the relations between money and giving. You cannot give money in the gratuitous sense of giving, because money is pure exchange. The gratuitous gift, as opposed to the reciprocating gift, requires that it is possible for the object that is given to remain forever with the person to whom it is given. There is a promise of eternity in this gift. Those aunts and uncles who give money as presents are perceived as wanting in something: in imagination. When a father gives his son a check for a birthday present, we sense a violation of the logic of the gift that is no less fundamental than when a son gives a check as a gift to his father. What is lacking here is exactly what is evoked by the notion of the pure gift as excess beyond—or before—exchange relations. Within Marxist theory, this is captured in the contrast of use-value and exchange-value: the residue that comes before or after exchange relations—the part that cannot be assimilated to exchange, that is only use or uselessness.

The psychoanalytic equivalences provide an ironic commentary on this logic of exchange and utility: feces = penis = baby. Feces are the exemplary useless object—although, as I have already indicated, their cooption into the circuit of exchange through the cyclical utopias of nineteenth-century sewage engineering, or through the rice growers of China buying human excrement at the gates of the city in order to transport it to the fields, is by no means uncommon. Similarly, at the other end of the circuit of life and of the body, the baby is exemplary of the object that cannot be exchanged, that is pure potential use-value prior to any possible use. When asked what use his lightning conductor would be, Benjamin Franklin replied: "What use is a baby?" There are objects, often the most prized, whose utility lies precisely in their lack of use and the promise of their inner transformation. Of the penis and the law of its exchange-value, I will have more to say later.

My concern with the inadequacies of the Maussian model and its development by Lévi-Strauss and Lacan is intriguingly highlighted by Fernand Braudel's consideration of the question of the place of the market in history.[84] He considers Karl Polanyi's Maussian view, that the circulation of goods and trade through "ceremonial exchange governed by the principle of *reciprocity*"[85] predominated over the law of the market until the nineteenth century, when the self-regulating price mechanism came to dominate the world. One must, according to this view, distinguish trade from the market, differentiate between the circulation conceived of as a total social fact and the circulation governed by the money-relations of the market. Almost as if he had in mind Lacan's revision of the Oedipus complex using structuralist analyses of kinship structures, Braudel replies:

> There is no law against introducing into a discussion of the "great transformation" of the nineteenth century such phenomena as the *potlatch* or *kula* (rather than say the very diversified trading organiza-tion of the seventeenth and eighteenth centuries). But it is rather like drawing on Lévi-Strauss's explanation of kinship ties to elucidate the rules governing marriage in Victorian England. Not the slightest effort has been made to tackle the concrete and diverse reality of history . . . Sociologists and economists in the past and anthropologists today have unfortunately accustomed us to their almost total indifference to his-tory. It does of course simplify their task.[86]

Instead of this ahistorical disjunction between gift-and-reciprocity-based societies and market-money economies, Braudel endorses the view that non-market exchange systems and exchanges for money have always existed side by side: "It would be more accurate to think of the market economy as being built up step by step. As Marcel

153

Mauss used to say, 'it was the societies of the Western world that turned man into an economic animal, in very recent times.' Not everyone is yet agreed of course on the exact sense of 'very recent.'"[87] This ironic comment concerning what "very recent" might mean— citing Mauss, whose theories he has just deprived of historical plausibility—gives a clear sense that Braudel thought that a pre-market society is something like that moment in the future when the State will wither away. The Maussian moment, like the Marxist moment, is outside history.

This does not prevent Braudel's own account, like those he criticizes, from positing an outside to the circulation of trade and the market. Alongside Braudel's historical vision of the triumphant ubiquity and protean flexibility of the market rides the consistent critique of the present, as is evident in the three-tier model he proposes. Beneath the market there lies "the lowest stratum of the non-economy, the soil into which capitalism thrusts its roots but which it can never really penetrate. This lowest layer remains an enormous one."[88] Let us call this, to anticipate a later argument, the simple barter economy. Then, above that stratum, comes that market economy whose infinitely variegated possibilities Braudel's work documents, with its horizontal communications between different markets and its automatic coordination of supply, demand, and prices. Above the market there is the modern system of the anti-market, characterized by imperialism and the manipulation of the market, "where the great predators roam and the law of the jungle operates. This—today as in the past, before and after the industrial revolution—is the real home of capitalism."[89] These two other non-market strata depart from the logic of reciprocity, exchange, and circulation.

Braudel's evocation of the lowest stratum of the non-economy points us toward an outside of the humming system of trade and circulation, just as the gift's logic requires such an outside. Within theoretical economics and economic anthropology, there is a name given to this outside: barter. The classical model of barter envisages the development of a division of labor and a system of bartering between social groups of objects, one of which eventually became the measure, the yardstick, and the medium for facilitating future exchanges: money. Barter is the prototype of exchange in that one agent's demand is matched perfectly to the other's; an exchange takes place between these two free, desiring subjects, after which they are quits.[90] From the point of view of the exchangist, reciprocating model of circulation, this transaction is not part of a system, and, most important, does not give rise to any consequences. Whether or not barter ever gave or gives rise to a system of monetary exchange, which anthropologists now doubt, it lacks a crucial feature necessary for circulation to begin: there is no residue after the transaction is completed. Of course, the farmer who trades potatoes for pigs could barter the pigs for jewelry. But the basic system of barter does postulate a demand for goods that is filled by the objects bartered, and it is the level of this demand, and nothing else, that fixes the rate of equivalence. To invoke a potential yardstick that would match potatoes, pigs, and jewelry would impose the monetary system, would include it already at the heart of barter. Thus barter, in order to *be* barter, must be characterized by this essential link between demand and goods.

To get a system of circulation going on the basis of barter, one could, of course, postulate an inherent desire for trade: a *Verkehrtrieb*, a trading drive. But one of the virtues of the Maussian theory is precisely that it avoids such a vicarious, superfluous—gratuitous—hypothesis. The total prestation of the gift is asymmetrical, in contrast to barter, and leaves one of the parties in a state of obligation at the end of the transaction. It is this residual obligation—this debt—that is the motor of circulation in the gift-economies. Gift-economies operate entirely within the framework of compulsion and obligation between social unequals or persons asymmetrical in relation to each other—in contrast, it is argued, to barter, where the symmetry of the transaction is linked to the freedom of the agents and the automatic closure that exchange entails.

This freedom of the agents in barter and the fact that they are quits at the end of the transaction capture two crucial elements of the notion of the gift as gratuitous: first, the sense that my giving a present should not, in order for my gift to be a gift, entail an obligation on the recipient's part. My giving is free—is not under an obligation—otherwise it is not a gift, but a duty. Second, the other's receiving entails no future to our relationship. After I have given my gift, the other is richer by the gift he has received and I am poorer by what I have given, but we are still quits. We can leave without residual obligation. Thus barter includes two elements that evade the impossibility of the gift that Derrida spells out.

This observation makes one wonder whether Mauss may not have been trading implicitly on these properties of barter when he discussed the gift as prestation, even though his theory is diametrically opposed to proposing barter as the fundamental social fact. His theory goes precisely in the opposite direction: toward the recognition of universal and ubiquitous obligation, toward the concept of society as a system of reciprocal obligations. In Maussian mood, Marilyn Strathern questions the common "supposition that one can regard gift exchange as somehow a version of commodity exchange . . . [Anthropologists' concerns with the interpretation of marriage transactions] remain dominated by the assumption that there is an intention to the system as a whole, namely to enable men to obtain women. The market analogy presumably endures because it speaks so directly and strongly to Western constructions."[91] Strathern here highlights the fact that gift exchange, like commodity exchange, is immediately subsumed under the overarching descriptive-normative category of the system of circulation. It is this concept of the system and the internal dynamic of the system as being circulation that has had such a hold on anthropologists, sociologists, and, I am suggesting, certain psychoanalysts. As Strathern's critique indicates, she also wishes to find some other way to characterize gift exchange than as part of a system. Freedom and non-consequentiality (the two elements supposed by barter) are the two elements that indicate how this is accomplished. But, as we immediately recognize, these two elements are also the ones generally held up as the virtues of money.

Barter does not have a very strong conceptual profile. Yet it has a particular interest for psychoanalysis because the barter model of sexual relations is often held up as an ideal. The woman's potatoes are exchanged against the man's pigs. Both parties go away satisfied, having given what they are prepared to lose and having sated completely their desires.[92] This model is sometimes known as "free love." The emphasis—the word "free"—is placed entirely upon the mutual exchanging of sexual pleasure between two free and equal parties, whose sole aim is satisfying their desires and who, at the end of the affair, are quits. An imagined complementarity of gender roles can be stitched or grafted onto this conception, and can be suggested as the motive for the larger structures of alliance and marriage, thus installing the barter conception of sexuality at the heart of the general relations of reciprocity and exchange. Men barter marriage for sex, and women barter sex for marriage.

To make this system work, the two agents who enter into the barter must not only be equals and be in a symmetrical position with respect to each other, but they must also conceive of each other as complementary. The goods that one has to exchange match exactly the goods that the other has. But the kinship structures that overlap the gift exchanges of the Maussian system clearly leave little room for such a model of sexual relations. The circle must not close as abruptly and completely as this. Even if such a model of sexual relations existed, it would be entirely recuperated by the stronger systemic logic of the gift as reciprocity, which, it should not be forgotten, in Lévi-Strauss's hands became entirely preoccupied with the exchange of women and goods in accordance with the same logic.

The complementary model of sexual relations is foreign to psychoanalysis, from Freud's conception of the single model of development out of polymorphous perversity, through his thesis that there is only one libido, which is masculine, to the radical asymmetry of

157

Lacan's theories of sexual difference. Thus we see one more reason why the logic of gift and exchange can be grafted so comfortably onto psychoanalytic theory. The logic of sexual relations for psychoanalysis is always the logic of the supplement, not the complement.[93] It is through the supplement that sexuality opens out, is disseminated, into broader social relations—most conventionally in the baby, most controversially in the penis, most graphically in the feces: "Faeces are the child's first *gift*, the first sacrifice on behalf of his affection, a portion of his own body which he is ready to part with, but only for the sake of some one he loves."[94] But, as Derrida has so often convincingly reminded us, this logic of the supplement also has two sides: the supplement that is a gift as gratuitous, as surplus, and the supplement that is intrinsic to the internal logic of the whole, the supplement that is caught in the logic of substitution and repetition. Once the feces are caught in this logic, the string of substitutions, of symbols as Melanie Klein and Hanna Segal call them,[95] is endless. The feces turn into that universal medium of the gift known as money.

There are, however, quiet moments in the development of psychoanalytic thought that do not conform to the gift as exchange and reciprocity model. Curiously enough, we have seen one of them already, in the central transferential scene with the Rat Man where his dream of Freud's daughter with cow dung for eyes converged with an interpretation that Freud had given, some seven years earlier, of one of his own dreams. Freud interpreted both his and the Rat Man's dream according to the phrase "for the sake of your *beaux yeux*." For the Rat Man, this meant that he intended to marry Freud's daughter for her money, not for love. And in Freud's own dream the central thoughts were the contrast between "selfish" and "unselfish," between "being in debt" and "without paying for it."[96] Freud's wish was that he for once be given something for nothing. This is as apt and accurate a characterization of what we mean by a gift as one can find. The psychoanalytic theory of love is thus the wish—and is a wish itself a supplement, a beyond of the logic of reality with its substitutions?—that one be given something for nothing. In Lacan's definition of love—love is the gift of something one does not have—we are to be given a nothing that is something.

It is this nothing that is something that tempts one to see another side to Lacan's theory of the Symbolic, a side which is not entirely captive to the logic of circulation of the signifier. The other side of Lacan's theory of the signifier is his theory of speech. Speech is granted quasi-magical powers: founding speech, as I have analyzed it elsewhere.[97] But this founding speech can always be recuperated by including it within speech act theory, which itself leads to a new quasi-magical dimension: that of faith or confidence—the faith I lodge in the other, the confidence that is inherent in and founds (how can it found that which it creates?) the promise, the contract. Yet, as we now see from the paradox of the gift, this magical power will always reappear elsewhere. In Maussian mode, we find it at the end of Lacan's Rome Discourse, when he evokes the response of Prajapâti, the god of thunder from the Bhrad-âranyaka Upanishad, to the exhortation: "Speak to us. 'Da,' replies Prajapâti. Three times he says 'Da,' and three times he queries whether he has been understood. The first meaning of Da is submission, the second, gift, and the third is grace."[98] Lacan thus ends his advice to analysts with a reminder of the other dimension of the gift of speech: gift as pure gift, as grace. It is precisely this notion of grace that Christianity developed as its name for the gift from God that is not exchangeable or transferable with another human being. Grace is the name for a gift relationship that is excluded from exchange relations. Such is the power of the concept of the gift that it is not even clear that it makes any sense to say that grace is in God's gift.

---

My exposition—or rather my clarification—of the Lacanian Symbolic and its debt leads inexorably to the conclusion that the signifier of signifiers, the signifier that designates the effects of the system, as Lacan describes Lévi-Strauss's zero signifier, is not *hau*, is not *mana*, is not the quantum, is not even the phallus, but is—money. Let me briefly indicate how this new version of the classical analogy between speech and money may clarify matters.[99]

Lacan used the Rat Man's debt to put together his revision of "the general anthropology derived from analytic doctrine."[100] With the concept of debt, Lacan had found something that would harmonize equally well with the theory of the lack—whether in its existential version (*manque-à-être*, lack-in-being) or in its erotic version (the lack of the phallus)—and with the theory of speech, exchange, and death which underpinned the revision of the psychoanalytic anthropology. The reading of Freud he gave that sustained this new anthropology was certainly idiosyncratic, one might even say retroactively effective:

> In establishing, in *The Interpretation of Dreams*, the Oedipus complex as the central motivation of the unconscious, he recognized this unconscious as the agency of the laws on which marriage alliance and kinship are based . . . it is essentially on sexual relations—by ordering them according to the law of preferential marriage alliances and forbidden relations—that the first combinatory for the exchanges of women between nominal lineages is based, in order to develop in an exchange of gifts and in an exchange of master-words the fundamental commerce and concrete discourse on which human societies are based.[101]

This combinatory of exchanges—of gifts, women, and words—is quite explicitly a fundamental departure from Freud's theory. And in the 1930s Lacan had explicitly recognized it as such: the model of one primal horde, transformed into a society through the inner logic of the murder of the primal father, had, Lacan sensed, included the key (neo-Hegelian, neo-Kojèvian) intuition that the father becomes a human father insofar as he is dead; however, *Totem and Taboo*'s model of social relations was not only historically but also conceptually implausible.[102] To replace the anthropology of the father's murder, the key term in Lacan's anthropology became that of exchange. There are elementary structures of lineages, secured by the dynamic reality of renewed and repeated exchange—of women, gifts, and words. And "the exchange that characterizes such a society has other foundations than the needs even to satisfy them, what has been called the gift 'as total social fact.'"[103]

The metaphysics of speech eventually came to underpin this system of exchange which embodied the overly formal Maussian theory of the gift as expressing an algebra of obligation and reciprocity. To found Lacan's more generalized anthropology for psychoanalysis, he turned to a theory of full speech, of the unconditional obligation and unconscious effects of every act of speech.[104] And in this theory of speech, we come back to our starting-point—the prerequisites of trust and of faith: the Good Faith of the Other invoked in the act of speech.[105] And the concept of debt also finds a natural home here; it is also a means by which Lacan brings into the circle of mediations the concept of death. As the epigraph at the opening of this essay indicates, as Freud's Shakespearean "thou owest Nature a death" suggests, the debt that over-trumps all others, the debt that Lacan implies all other debts reduce to, in a ghostly and no doubt eternal circulation of debt, is the debt of death. We owe our lives to the dead father.

This is an attempt to establish a medium of symbolic exchange for Lacan's concept of the Symbolic. The unit of account is the tautologous debt, counted out by and measured against death. Yet this attempt to find the unit of currency of symbolic debt in death is not entirely convincing. First, this currency demands illumination by our more familiar practices associated with money—what we usually call the banking system. How revealing is the analogy with the banking system? In financial reality, when we hold money, when it sits in our wallets or gets sweaty between our fingers, it is the Bank that is in *our* debt. The confidence we have in the Bank is a way of saying we actually believe the Bank when it promises that it will honor the debt represented by the banknote; it will never foreclose on that debt. The modern banking system works in large part because the social roles of creditor and debtor have become refined to the point where "the debtor has become perfectly specific (in the guise of the state) and the creditor, completely general (in the guise of anyone who happens to have had the debt assigned to him). No one can be substituted for the debtor; anyone can be substituted for the creditor."[106] It is this feature, this extreme asymmetry in the relation between the ultimate debtor, the Bank, which is the starting-point and ultimate end-point in the circulation of money, and the ultimate creditor, who can only ever be the medium for the circulation of money, which makes it plausible to align it with the living and the dead.

It is true that money is well adapted to serve as the symbol of both life and death. As Simmel writes:

> There is no more striking symbol of the completely dynamic character of the world than that of money. The meaning of money lies in the fact that it will be given away. When money stands still, it is no longer money according to its specific value and significance. The effect that it occasionally exerts in a state of repose arises out of an anticipation of its further motion. Money is nothing but the vehicle for a movement in which everything else that is not in motion is completely extinguished. It is, as it were, an *actus purus;* it lives in continuous self-alienation from any given point and thus forms the counterpart and direct negation of all being in itself.[107]

When money stops moving, it dies, it becomes being in itself, that is, death. When it returns to the Bank, to the Treasury (of signifiers), it dies. The Bank is thus, as we all know from the iconography of our culture over the last few centuries, the place from which all economic life emanates—it is the place of death. We stopped building mausoleums because the banks, built in their image, came to serve that function of housing the most socially essential of our dead. The Bank is that exemplary institution for attempting to refute the adage that you can't take it with you.

But we should also take a step back in the argument. To talk of debt, we must be in the realm of the countable. We must always be able to ask: "How *much* is owed?" We should take our argument from another Hegelian, Karl Marx:

> This commodity [exchange value] is the commodity as money, and, to be precise, not as money in general, but as a *certain definite sum of money*, for, in order to represent exchange value in all its variety, money has to be countable, quantitatively divisible. Money—the common form into which all commodities as exchange values are transformed, i.e. the universal commodity—must itself exist as a *particular* commodity alongside the others, since what is required is not only that they can be measured against it in the head, but that they can be changed and exchanged for it in the actual exchange process.[108]

We can take our cue from the Rat Man: he knew *exactly* how much he owed Lieutenant A. Freud's text repeats the figure on numerous occasions: 3.80 kronen. But, as Freud and Lacan are both aware, this is his imaginary debt. His symbolic debt may well have been, may have had to have been, countable in a different currency. So what is the currency of Lacan's symbolic debt?

Lacan's social theory vacillates on this point. Is he committed to the view that debt is measured in terms of a substance, like coins or papers? Or does he view debt as an accounting procedure, a system of writing which records the transactions of the parties?[109] We might view his later explorations of number theory as one way to answer this question. The theory of the *trait unaire* (unique or single trait) of his Seminars in the early 1960s, together with the theory of suture elaborated by Jacques-Alain Miller, would thus be attempts at rendering Lévi-Strauss's theory of the zero-signifier into a properly countable theory of symbolic debt.[110] If this is the case, it would seem that Lacan's theory always leaned toward the accounting procedure— toward the notion that debt is given by a mark, a piece of writing, like the first system of money of which we have records, the Sumerian bricks upon which marks register debts.

As we have seen, the balance of the metaphors and figures that Lacan employs following Lévi-Strauss and Mauss is toward the movement of women, objects, and signifiers, a movement which reflects the inverse movement at the unconscious level of debt. But the emphasis on the good faith of the other, whether in reciprocal exchange or in speech, prompted Lacan to introduce the concept of the Big Other, and therein lay part of his conceptual ingenuity—the combining and interleaving of the discourses of philosophy, linguistics, and ethnology. The Big Other began to function somewhat like a bank—the treasury of signifiers, as Lacan called it. The notorious indefiniteness of Lacan's concept of the Other includes among its many other functions this financial function, of upholding the system of debt, of keeping it from folding in a crisis of confidence, which the symbolic father creates. And we also know the element that functions as some kind of guarantee of the system: it is known as the phallus, the gold standard of the system of symbolic debt. This is one of the bridges to the psychoanalytic theory of sexuality: the phallus is the key term by which the notion of symbolic debt is rendered workable in clinical accounts of sexuality. The phallus very neatly conforms to another of the properties of money that Marx noted,[111] that of allowing "the equation of the incompatible, as Shakespeare nicely defined money: 'Thou visible God! / That solder'st close impossibilities, / And mak'st them kiss!'"[112] In exactly parallel fashion, the phallus acts, as a famously controversial passage from Lacan asserts, by joining "la part du logos" to "l'avènement du désir" (the side of logos to the coming of desire):

> It can be said that this signifier is chosen because it is the most tangible element in the real of sexual copulation, and also the most symbolic in the literal (typographical) sense of the term, since it is equivalent to the (logical) copula. It might also be said that, by virtue of its turgidity, it is the image of the vital flow as it is transmitted in generation.[113]

It is by now a notorious and, for many people, a risible aspect of Lacanian theory that its practitioners and theorists are obliged to engage in neo-scholastic disquisitions on the distinction between the phallus and the penis. The implications of the distinction are most easily seen, I would argue, by comparing it to that between money and gold. Gold, like the penis, has a long, distinguished, and venerable history as the unique marker of value. Yet all economic theorists since Marx, and all bankers since the 1930s, accept that the relation between money and gold is a contingent one. We can write a history of gold that encompasses its relations with luxury, empire, mining, and colonialism, in which the desire for gold sweeps over whole cultures, transforming history—whether in the pogroms of South America or the Gold Rushes of Alaska, South Africa, and California—through to the psychotic identification of gold and wealth. The entire technology of mining in Europe, and thus the technology that introduced the steam engine into the economy, depends, according to Nef and Braudel, upon the commerce in silver of the early modern period. And out of this fetishism of gold and silver emerges modern money, which repudiates its kinship to gold, expels the figure of gold into the outer darkness of theatrical comedy and the nineteenth-century novel by creating the unforgettably sad portrait of the miser. The miser is the realist of money, overtaken by the money revolution, which introduces the dialectic of negativity into all social relations; as Keynes put it, "it is a recognized characteristic of money as a store of wealth that it is barren; whereas practically every other form of storing wealth yields some interest or profit. Why should anyone outside a lunatic asylum wish to use money as a store of wealth?"[114] Money is the negation of all other goods; it is the means through which all other goods acquire value; it is the universal medium and also the universal standard, which can only be quantified in its movement, not in its accumulation.

The contentious relation of the body's organs to the phallus can thus, I suggest, be best thought of as akin to the relation of gold to money. Having insisted on this link between the signifier of value and the circulation that constitutes the Symbolic, Lacan cashes out this theory when he addresses the relations between the sexes:

> The symbolic parity *Mädchen* = *Phallus* [girl = phallus] . . . has its root
> in the imaginary paths by which the child's desire succeeds in identi-
> fying itself with the mother's want-to-be, to which of course she was
> herself introduced by the symbolic law in which this lack is consti-
> tuted.
>
> It is as a result of the same mechanism that women in the real order
> serve, if they'll forgive me saying so, as objects for the exchanges
> required by the elementary structures of kinship and which are some-
> times perpetuated in the imaginary order, while what is transmitted in
> a parallel way in the symbolic order is the phallus.[115]

Lacan also sensed that a system of exchange, of money, may not
be an entirely stable self-regulating system; it may require something
outside of itself to maintain it. Money often attaches itself to other
social institutions (for example, the state as guaranteed by its military
power) for this stabilizing function, which can never fully escape from
the paradoxes associated with good faith. As Crump remarks, "the
dominant political factor relating to the manufacture of money is the
need to maintain confidence, which in turn requires that what comes
from certain recognized producers as money is certified as genuine."[116] Just like the Bank, Lacan may have felt that the reference to
the good faith, the confidence, of the creditors suffices only up to a
point. Even Lacan was not immune to the realization that faith in the
phallus is not unlimited, and that another principle may be required
to sustain it when questions about its right of hegemony are raised:

> The law would not apply any the less if women were placed at the
> centre of this system, receiving the phallus in exchange for which they
> would give a child. If one must however describe this exchange as
> androcentric, it is, Lévi-Strauss tells us, on account of effects which
> make themselves felt, of political power that it is incumbent on men
> to exercise. The phallus prevails, then, because it is also the sceptre,
> in other words because it belongs to the symbolic order.[117]

Yet, despite the undoubted analogy between the precious substances
for so long associated with money and the relation of the penis and

the phallus, there is no means of measuring symbolic debt. This is not to say that counting and measuring are excluded from an individual subject's relations to the penis; far from it. But every attempt to turn the penis into a countable measure of value is, in the end, as eccentric as the Rat Man measuring his debt in rats. Such attempts are closely akin to those which seek the most precious word in the language, for instance in the search for magic words or, more successfully, in poetry. Perhaps we might conclude that the currency in which the symbolic debt is counted will be unique to each and every analytic subject. The rat currency of the Rat Man will have to remain our model, through which we look beyond his imaginary commerce to the symbolic debt he owed his father, which can only be recognized through the mediation of his death.

———

There is a lesson in psychoanalytic technique to be drawn from the question of the countability of the symbolic debt. We have seen how Freud was quite clear that he would not get drawn into the system of imaginary debts the Rat Man was caught in, and I have drawn attention to the fact that Lacan, mistakenly, implicated Freud more closely in that system than Freud's own account warrants. Freud did not respond to the demand of the Rat Man for a medical certificate to aid his payment of the debt which still haunted him. But, no matter how well the analyst steers clear of imaginary involvement, there is the by no means simple question of extricating oneself from the transference.

Lacan argued that it is money that neutralizes the effects of the transference. In the end, then, it looks as if the imaginary debts of the patient—which are all translated into imaginary debts to the analyst—can be translated into the Symbolic and counted out in notes, checks, credit card accounts, futures options, paintings, or whatever else is transacted between patient and analyst. This is, as everyone is aware, a sensitive topic. Freud recognized that, for a number of reasons, it is essential that psychoanalysis be made countable. "Free treatment enormously increases some of a neurotic's resistances—in young women, for instance, the temptation which is inherent in their transference-relation, and in young men, their opposition to an obligation to feel grateful . . . The absence of the regulating effect offered by the payment of a fee to the doctor makes itself very painfully felt."[118] Freud also emphasized that "civilized people" treat money matters with the same inconsistency, hypocrisy, and prudishness as they do the sexual. The sense in which this may lead to incongruous effects can be gauged from Ferenczi's story of a patient who opened a consultation by saying: "'Doctor, if you help me, I'll give you every penny I possess!' 'I shall be satisfied with thirty kronen an hour,' the physician replied. 'But isn't that rather excessive?' the patient unexpectedly remarked."[119]

The well-regulated analysis will, then, manage to match the transference with the analytic fee in an equilibrated system where obligation, reciprocation, and service are perfectly aligned. This vision is the small-scale counterpart of Lacan's grand vision of the circulating symbolic debt. This is the ideal of a perfect circulation, with no dead letters, where no letters or checks go astray. The letters arrive at their destination, as if they did indeed form part of a great *kula*. But if the vision of the circulation of debt and obligation in Melanesia took on a heroic hue for Malinowski, who cast his social actors as the Argonauts of the Western Pacific, within the analytic consulting-room this vision of finely equilibrated circulation is recognizably an obsessional world of circulation and debt, in which every death is replaced by a new life, so as to keep the stranger at the door. Lacan's theory of debt is a theory of social life as obsessional in structure. The universality of debt may well be based on a gratuitous assumption, akin to the Beatles' declamatory: "And in the end, the love you take is equal to the love you make." What if social life isn't like that? What if social life is more chaotic and unregulated than that? What if there are myriad unintended consequences, myriad superfluous actions and wild movements that introduce novelty? What if the other side of the concept of gift, its surprising gratuity, its capacity to create something out of nothing, is also inescapably active, both in the social and the psychoanalytic worlds? What if lying, which shares with the gift its gratuity and its instantaneous disruption of the circulation of honest words and things, is also an essential principle of creative innovation, wiping out debt and wreaking havoc with the Symbolic's accounting system? What if psychoanalysis, despite itself, allows the possibility of something new happening, something that is not a repetition?

As Derrida noted very pointedly in his reading of the "Seminar on *The Purloined Letter*," Lacan follows Freud's lead in seeing money as the means of neutralizing transference. In Lacan's allegorical reading of Poe's story, the large check Dupin receives is the equivalent to the analytic fee. "Is this the way that the debt finally gets paid off? If symbolic efficacity stops there [with the finding and the return of the purloined letter to the Prefect], is that because the symbolic debt is also extinguished there?"[120] Here, at last, when the speaking stops, at the end of analysis, appears the signifier of signifiers. And, you might reflect, it is better for analysts to be paid in money than in phalluses—though one might be somewhat surprised by the extent to which analytic efficacy is measured in babies. What indeed would happen if analysts were paid in kind, if Freud really had been paid in rats?

Lacan shows that it is not so easy for Dupin to extract himself from the letter's symbolic circuit; such a thought might have been one reason why he implicated Freud further in the Rat Man's system of debt than he had himself recognized. Two incidents in Poe's story demonstrate this: first, the infernal trap Dupin leaves for the Minister, with the deadly lines from Crébillon. This, as Lacan indicates, and as Derrida underlines in his commentary "Le facteur de la vérité," shows how Dupin does not extract himself successfully. Does the other incident—Dupin's demand for an extremely large fee—make the termination of the system of obligations and debts of analysis any more likely?

Does this mean that this Dupin, who up until then was an admirable, almost excessively lucid character, has all of a sudden become a small time wheeler and dealer? I don't hesitate to see in this action the re-purchasing of what one could call the bad *mana* attached to the letter. And indeed, from the moment he receives his fee, he has pulled out of the game. It isn't only because he has handed the letter over to another, but because his motives are clear to everyone—he got his money, it's no longer of any concern to him.

I don't mean to insist on it, but you might gently point out to me that we, who spend our time being the bearers of all the purloined letters of the patient, also get paid somewhat dearly. Think about this with some care—were we not to be paid, we would get involved in the drama of Atreus and Thyestes, the drama in which all the subjects who come to confide their truth in us are involved. They tell us all their damned [*sacré*] stories, and because of that we are not at all within the domain of the sacred and of sacrifice. Everyone knows that money doesn't just buy things, but that the prices which, in our culture, are calculated at rock-bottom, have the function of neutralising something infinitely more dangerous than paying in money, namely owing somebody something.[121]

In truth, this does not seem a very reliable method for extracting oneself from the system of symbolic debt. It may take more than money for the analyst to step outside of the system of imaginary circulation of debt. Dupin's actions are a model here, with their gratuitous spite and venom. Nor is it superfluous to recall how gratuitous and unpredictable were Lacan's own practices when it came to analytic fees.

And this dangerous situation of owing something to somebody reminds us that, in the end, it is not clear if Lacan as a reader of Freud owes more to Freud than Freud owes to Lacan, to posterity, and any given reader whatsoever. After all, if symbolic debt is countable and commutative, then the dead are in credit to posterity.

———

There is one phrase from Freud's letters to Fliess concerning money which has been repeatedly quoted by commentators, as if it supplies its own interpretation. While writing his Dreckology, his Shitology,

to his Berlin friend, Freud opined: "Happiness is the belated fulfil-
ment of a prehistoric wish. For this reason wealth brings so little
happiness. Money was not a childhood wish."[122] When he made this
discovery, Freud was up to his arms in the fantasy material that would
later become his theory of the anal phase, on which the famous
equation of money and excrement was built. But more to my point
here is the fact that he was engaged in finally detaching himself from
his friendship with Breuer, attempting to pay off his debts to him—
2,300 florins, to be precise. The story had, by 1898, become very
complicated for Freud, since Breuer refused to accept Freud's payment of his old debt, incurred in the early 1880s when Freud was an
impoverished student. However, by 1898, Breuer thought he was
indebted to Freud, who had analyzed a relative of his over a period
of some years. Freud was furious at not being allowed to pay off his
debt; but Breuer's actions also provoked another reaction in Freud.
Breuer was in the habit of criticizing Freud for not saving enough:
he went on too many holidays, and his new hobby of collecting
antiquities was an expensive one. Freud's dream of the Botanical
Monograph, which occurred a few weeks later, was a direct response
to Breuer's refusal to accept the repayment of the debt. Freud
discovered that the wish informing the dream was for permission to
indulge his hobbies, his whims, his desires.[123]

There is no doubt that Freud wished to clear his account, to pay
off that debt to Breuer, just as Lacan tried to clear his account with
Freud. But it may be no accident that this was the very moment in
his life when Freud found a place in his theoretical system for the
"discovery" that money can never make you happy. When I was
younger, I was very struck by a comment in a conversation where my
interlocutor described a mutual close friend as having a gift for being
happy. Perhaps that is what Freud's discovery that infantile wishes
are foreign to the logic of money—and the entire logic of debt,
exchange, and reciprocity—amounted to: that our deepest wishes are
for something that is as gratuitous, as full of grace, as happiness. The
gift of something for nothing.

171

ABBREVIATIONS

NOTES

ACKNOWLEDGMENTS

INDEX

# ABBREVIATIONS

*E*              Jacques Lacan, *Ecrits* (Paris: Seuil, 1966). Where a second figure is given it refers to the English translation, *Ecrits: A Selection*, trans. Alan Sheridan (London: Tavistock/New York: Norton, 1977). Where a reference is given solely to the English translation, the page number will be followed by (Engl.)

*FF*             *The Complete Letters of Sigmund Freud to Wilhelm Fliess, 1887–1904*, ed. J. M. Masson (Cambridge, Mass.: Harvard University Press, 1984)

*ID*             Sigmund Freud, *The Interpretation of Dreams*, Vols. IV and V of *SE*

*Int. J. Psa.*   *International Journal of Psycho-analysis*

*SE*             Sigmund Freud, *The Standard Edition of the Complete Psychological Works of Sigmund Freud*, 24 vols., edited by James Strachey in collaboration with Anna Freud, assisted by Alix Strachey and Alan Tyson (London: The Hogarth Press and the Institute of Psycho-analysis, 1953–1974)

*Stud*           Sigmund Freud, *Studienausgabe*, 10 vols. with an unnumbered *Ergänzungsband* (abbreviated as *Erg*) (Frankfurt am Main: Fischer Verlag, 1969–1975)

# NOTES

## Introduction

1. Michel Foucault introduced the notion of "truth games" in the last of his writings; there is also an obvious and helpful analogy with Wittgenstein's language games.

2. Harold J. Berman, *Law and Revolution: The Formation of the Western Legal Tradition* (Cambridge, Mass.: Harvard University Press, 1983).

3. For two recent and instructive accounts, see Patricia Kitcher, *Freud's Dream: A Complete Interdisciplinary Science of the Mind* (Cambridge, Mass.: MIT Press, 1992), and E. Fuller Torrey, *Freudian Fraud: The Malignant Effect of Freud's Theory on American Thought and Culture* (New York: HarperCollins, 1992). The maritime metaphor is borrowed from Mary Douglas, for whom psychoanalytic theory is "too much like a ship at anchor, once fitted out for a great voyage, but sails now furled, ropes flapping, motion stilled. It is not as if theoretical winds were lacking to drive it. But the motive to go somewhere is missing." Mary Douglas, *In the Active Voice* (London: RKP, 1982), p. 14.

## Truth Games

### I: Knowing Lies

1. Augustine, *De mendacio* (On Lying) (395), in *Treatise on Various Subjects*, ed. R. J. Deferrari, Fathers of the Church, vol. 16 (New York: Fathers of the Church, 1952), pp. 51–110, and *Contra mendacium* (Against Lying) (420), in ibid., vol. 16, pp. 121–179.

2. Cutting across this theme is another: the relation of present to future. In Hebraic thought, prophecy is always contingent upon God's will, so that what is prophesied will come to pass because God has written it, and will therefore realize it. If He withdraws His hand, if He changes His mind, the prophetic relation to the future lapses. In Greek thought, on the other hand, what the oracle says will always come to pass—the problem resides in the ambiguity of

the oracle's words, and the difficulties of interpretation that result. Hence the dialectic of appearance and reality reappears in another familiar guise: that of deciphering. What is deciphered correctly *is* the future.

3. Jean-Paul Sartre, *Being and Nothingness: A Phenomenological Essay on Ontology* (1943), trans. Hazel E. Barnes (New York: Philosophical Library, 1956), see in particular pp. 86–95; this passage from p. 88.

4. See Maxime Chastaing, "Connaissez-vous les uns les autres?" in *Psychologie comparative et art: Hommage à I. Meyerson* (Paris: Presses Universitaires de France, 1972), pp. 255–264.

5. Vladimir Jankélévitch, *Du mensonge,* 2nd ed. (Lyon: Saint-Amand-Montrand, 1945; 1st ed., 1940), p. 21.

6. Friedrich Nietzsche, *Das Philosophenbuch* (1873), Part III, "Knowledge-theoretical Introduction on Truth and Lies in an Extra-moral Sense" (Paris: Aubier Flammarion Bilingue, 1969), p. 172 (my translation); see the English translation in Nietzsche, *Philosophy and Truth: Selections from Nietzsche's Notebooks of the Early 1870s,* trans. and ed. with Introduction and Notes by Daniel Breazeale (Atlantic Highlands, N.J.: Humanities/Hassocks, Sussex: Harvester, 1979), p. 80.

7. Karl Popper, "Karl Popper, Replies to My Critics," in *The Philosophy of Karl Popper,* ed. Paul Arthur Schilpp (La Salle, Ill.: Open Court, 1974), pp. 1112–1113; emphasis in the original. See George Steiner, *After Babel: Aspects of Language and Translation* (Oxford: Oxford University Press, 1975), p. 224.

8. That truth is primarily a moral question was argued by Rousseau: "My professed truthfulness is based more on feelings of integrity and justice than on factual truth, and I have been guided in practice more by the moral dictates of my conscience than by abstract notions of truth and falsehood. I have often made up stories, but very rarely told lies." Jean-Jacques Rousseau, *Reveries of the Solitary Walker* (1777), trans. Peter France (Harmondsworth: Penguin, 1979), "Fourth Walk," p. 79. See also p. 80, where truth-telling becomes a consequence of the requirements of justice: "If one must act justly towards others, one must act truthfully towards oneself. Truth is an homage that the good man pays to his own dignity."

9. See Bruno Latour, "Visualization and Cognition: Thinking with Eyes and Hands," *Knowledge and Society: Studies in the Sociology of Culture Past and Present* 6 (1986): 1–40, and John Forrester, "Dead on Time," in Forrester, *The Seductions of Psychoanalysis: Freud, Lacan, and Derrida* (Cambridge: Cambridge University Press, 1990), pp. 168–218.

10. For a detailed account of how truth was generated in seventeenth-century England, see Steven Shapin, *A Social History of Truth: Civility and Science in Seventeenth Century England* (Chicago: University of Chicago Press, 1994).

11. Leopold Infeld, *Quest: The Evolution of a Scientist* (London: Readers Union/Victor Gollancz, 1942), p. 215. Infeld gives the contemporary American version of "Rafiniert ist Herr Gott aber boshaft ist Er nicht" as "God is slick but He ain't mean," which Norbert Wiener also follows; but, as I point out later in the essay, Wiener makes completely explicit the intentionally deceptive connotations of *boshaft*.

12. Quoted in Holton, "On the Psychology of Scientists and Their Social Concerns," in Gerald Holton, *The Scientific Imagination: Case Studies* (Cambridge: Cambridge University Press, 1978), pp. 231–232.

13. For a general introduction to these, see Sissela Bok, *Lying: Moral Choice in Public and Private Life* (Hassock, Sussex: Harvester, 1978), which includes a useful bibliography and excerpts from classic texts. Other works on lying that I have found particularly useful include those by Augustine and Nietzsche cited in the text; Oscar Wilde's *The Decay of Lying;* Vladimir Jankélévitch, *Du mensonge;* and Jean-Paul Sartre, *Being and Nothingness.*

14. See also Kenneth Burke, *The Rhetoric of Religion: Studies in Logology* (Berkeley: University of California Press, 1970).

15. It also includes an intriguing argument based on a consideration of Jesus' injunction to "Love thy neighbor as thyself": "If a person sacrifices his own temporal life for the temporal life of another, he no longer loves the other as himself, but more than himself, and thus he exceeds the regulation of sound doctrine. Much less, then, may he, by lying, lose his eternal life for the temporal life of another" (*De mendacio,* p. 67).

16. For further details, see Louis Duchesne, *Early History of the Catholic Church,* trans. Claude Jenkins (London, 1914–1924), 3 vols., vol. 2, pp. 418–435, and vol. 3, pp. 404–406, and E.-Ch. Babut, *Priscillian et le Priscillianisme* (Paris, 1909).

17. Augustine, *Contra mendacium,* p. 130.

18. There is more than a hint in Augustine's arguments of the form of decision theory argument to be found first clearly expounded in Pascal's wager and to be so influential in the twentieth century.

19. And others, for example the Priscillianist view that the soul partakes of the same nature as God. For Augustine, this was blasphemy, since it indicated that God was subject to change and corruption.

20. This view was somewhat adapted in Kant's later writings, with the introduction of the categorical imperative, in which the category of "humanity" is more immediately covered by the famous argument concerning willing that a maxim become a universal law; see Immanuel Kant, *Groundwork of the Metaphysic of Morals,* trans. H. J. Paton (New York: Harper and Row, 1964), p. 70; but the criterion of treating humanity always as an end as well as a means is

introduced subsequently (see p. 96). For a contemporary exposition of this position, see Isaiah Berlin, *Four Essays on Liberty* (Oxford: Clarendon Press, 1968), especially "Two Concepts of Liberty" (1957), pp. 118–138.

21. Kant, "On a Supposed Right to Lie from Altruistic Motives" (1797), in *Critique of Practical Reason and Other Writings in Moral Philosophy*, ed. and trans. Lewis White Beck (Chicago: University of Chicago Press, 1949), pp. 346–350; see the discussion in Bok, *Lying*, p. 38. In 1786 he had been a little more flexible on the question. Certain lies are admissible: namely, those told to children and madmen. Passing over the madmen, why did Kant feel that one had a right to lie to children? Children, prompted by curiosity, Kant argued, ask questions such as "Where do babies come from?" In such a circumstance, "one can satisfy them easily in giving them absurd replies, which signify nothing, or in deflecting them by saying that that sort of question is childish." See Immanuel Kant, *Réflexions sur l'éducation* (1776–1787), trans. and introduction by A. Philonenko (Paris: Vrin, 1966); Kant, *Lectures on Ethics*, trans. Louis Infeld (London: Methuen, 1930); and the discussion in Dominique Colas, "Mensonge péda-gogique et sexualité enfantine chez Kant," *Ornicar?* 2 (1975): 73–75.

22. Voltaire to Thierot, 28 October 1736, in Theodore Besterman, ed., *Voltaire: Correspondence*, vol. IV–V (Geneva: Institut et Musée Voltaire, 1954), pp. 286–287.

23. Sir E. Thomas Browne, *Pseudodoxia epidemica*, in *Works*, vol. 2 (London: Faber, 1964), p. 76, quoted in J. A. Barnes, "The Importance of Lying," un-published paper, University of Cambridge, August 1983, and also in Barnes, "Lying: A Sociological View," *Australian Journal of Forensic Sciences* 15 (1983): 153; see also Samuel Johnson, *Selected Essays from the Rambler, Adventurer, and Idler*, ed. W. J. Bate (London and New Haven: Yale University Press, 1976), chap. 3.

24. David Bloor, *Knowledge and Social Imagery* (1976), 2nd ed. (Chicago: University of Chicago Press, 1991).

25. Alexandre Koyré, "Réflexions sur le mensonge," in *Renaissance* (New York: Ecole libre des hautes études, 1943), I (1943), pp. 95–111; this passage is from p. 95.

26. Ibid., p. 102.

27. Ibid., p. 104.

28. Hugh Hartshorne and Mark Arthur May, *Studies in the Nature of Char-acter*, 3 vols. (New York: Macmillan, 1928), vol. 1, p. 19.

29. David Hume, *An Enquiry concerning the Principles of Morals*, in L. A. Selby-Bigge, ed., *Enquiries concerning Human Understanding and Concerning the Principles of Morals*, 3rd ed., with text revised and notes by P. H. Nidditch (Oxford: Clarendon Press, 1975), pp. 282–283.

30. Oliver Wendell Holmes, Jr., "The Path of the Law" (1897), in *The Essential Holmes: Selections from the Letters, Speeches, Judicial Opinions, and Other Writings of Oliver Wendell Holmes, Jr.*, ed. Richard Posner (Chicago and London: University of Chicago Press, 1992), pp. 160–177.

31. Friedrich Nietzsche, *Daybreak: Thoughts on the Prejudices of Morality*, trans R. J. Hollingdale, introduction by Michael Tanner (Cambridge: Cambridge University Press, 1982), para. 306, p. 156.

32. Jankélévitch, *Du mensonge*, p. 19. See also Plato, *Lesser Hippias* 366d–367c, in which Socrates persuades a sophist that he who is most competent to speak truly about an issue is also the most competent to speak falsely about that issue—the exemplars of truth and falsity are Achilles and Odysseus. There are parallel arguments in the *Republic* I 333e.

33. Shakespeare, *As You Like It*, V.4.104–105.

34. J. Aitchison, *The Articulate Mammal: An Introduction to Psycholinguistics* (London: Unwin Hyman, 1989), p. 5.

35. See Richard Dawkins, *The Selfish Gene*, 2nd ed. (New York and Oxford: Oxford University Press, 1989), pp. 64–65 and p. 77, where Dawkins notes: "In the war of attrition, telling lies is no more evolutionarily stable than telling the truth. The poker face is evolutionarily stable."

36. Friedrich Nietzsche, *The Will to Power*, trans. Walter Kaufmann and R. J. Hollingdale (New York: Vintage, 1968), para. 378, p. 204.

37. "J'ai toujours vu que si l'on se mettait une seule minute à dire ce que l'on pensait, la société s'écroulerait."

38. Jankélévitch, *Du mensonge*, p. 33.

39. Shakespeare, Sonnet 138.

40. Marcel Proust, *Remembrance of Things Past*, vol. 1, trans C. K. Scott Moncrieff and Terence Kilmartin (London: Penguin, 1983), p. 544.

41. R. L. Stevenson, "Truth of Intercourse," Part IV of *Virginibus Puerisque*, in *Virginibus Puerisque and other essays in Belles Lettres* (1881) (London: William Heinemann, 1924), pp. 30–38; this quote is from p. 35.

42. Shere Hite, *The Hite Report on Female Sexuality* (1976) (London: Pandora, 1989), p. 262.

43. Hume, *Enquiry*, ed. Selby-Bigge, p. 200.

44. Quoted in Bok, *Lying*, p. 47.

45. Proust, *Remembrance of Things Past*, vol. 1, p. 1000.

46. Jonathan Swift, *A Tale of a Tub* (1704), 2nd ed., ed. A. C. Guthkelch and D. Nichol Smith (Oxford: Clarendon Press, 1958), section IX, pp. 172–173.

47. Proust, *Remembrance of Things Past*, vol. 3, p. 213.

48. J. M. Keynes, "The Commemoration of Thomas Robert Malthus. The Allocutions III. Mr Keynes," *Economic Journal* (June 1935), reprinted in *Essays*

*in Biography* in *Collected Writings of J. M. Keynes* (London: Macmillan for the Royal Economic Society, 1972), vol. 10, p. 106.

49. For work on the importance of deception in recent cognitive psychological accounts of autism, see U. Frith, J. Morton, and A. M. Leslie, "The Cognitive Basis of a Biological Disorder: Autism," *Trends in Neuroscience* 14 (1991): 433–438; B. Sodian and U. Frith, "Deception and Sabotage in Autistic, Retarded, and Normal Children," *Journal of Child Psychology and Psychiatry* 33 (1992): 591–605; S. Baron-Cohen, "The Development of a Theory of Mind in Autism: Deviance and Delay?" in M. Konstantareas and J. Beitchman, eds., *Psychiatric Clinics of North America* 14 (1991): 33–51. An excellent summary of this work can be found in Simon Baron-Cohen, *Mindblindness: An Essay on Autism and Theory of Mind* (Cambridge and London: MIT Press, 1995).

50. J. Gabel, *La Fausse Conscience: Essai sur la Réification* (Paris: Minuit, 1962), p. 127.

51. Ingmar Bergman, *The Magic Lantern: An Autobiography*, trans. Joan Tate (London: Penguin, 1988), pp. 9–12.

52. Jankélévitch, *Du mensonge*, p. 14. The French term *conscience* is translated both by "consciousness" and by "conscience." Jankélévitch continues (p. 15): "One will perhaps find, in looking close enough, that the eternal theme of feminine perfidy translates in its way this deception of reflective man, 'conscius sibi, secum exsistens,' who failed to find in her company the indivisibility [*l'indivision*] of his original *naïveté."*

53. Michel de Montaigne, "On the Cannibals," in *The Essays of Michel de Montaigne*, trans. and ed. with an introduction and notes by M. A. Screech (London: Allen Lane/Penguin Press, 1991), pp. 233–236.

54. Ten Rhyne, "The Journal of Ten Rhyne," in I. Schapera, ed., *The Early Cape Hottentot*, VRS 14 (Cape Town, 1933), p. 123, and G. Grevenbrock, *An Elegant Account of the African Race* (1695), p. 173. I owe these references to Rooha Variava, "The Deployment of Racism in South Africa," Ph.D. dissertation, University of Cambridge, 1989.

55. See K. L. Schäfer, "Kommen Lügen bei den Kindern vor dem vierten Jahre vor?" *Zeitschrift für pädagog. Psychol.* 7 (1905): 195–201; the question is discussed at length in Otto Lipmann and Paul Plaut, eds., *Die Lüge* (Leipzig: Barth, 1927), and in W. Stern and C. Stern, *Erinnerung, Aussage und Lüge in der ersten Kindheit* (Leipzig: J. A. Barth, 1931).

56. Joseph H. Smith, "The First Lie," *Psychiatry* 31 (1968): 61–68.

57. Jean Paul, quoted in Josef Spieler, *Le Petit Menteur* (Avignon: E. Aubanel, 1955), p. 9.

58. David Hume, *A Treatise of Human Nature* (1739–1740) (Harmondsworth: Penguin, 1969), book I, part 3, sec. 10, p. 170.

59. Hjalmar Frisk, "'Wahrheit' und 'Lüge' in der indogermanischen Sprachen, einige morphologischen Beobachtungen," *Göteborg Högskolas Arsskrift* 41 (1935): 1–39 (Göteborg: Elanders boktryckeri aktiebolag, 1936), esp. pp. 32–33.

60. From Emily Dickinson, "Tell all the Truth but tell it slant."

61. Freud, *Group Psychology and the Analysis of the Ego, SE* XVIII, 136–137.

62. Homer, *Iliad,* 9.308 et seq.

63. Plato, *Lesser Hippias* 364c–365d.

64. Nietzsche, *The Will to Power,* para. 495, p. 272.

65. Nietzsche, "Uber Wahrheit und Lüge," p. 174; "On Truth and Lies," p. 81.

66. Ibid.

67. Ibid., p. 178; p. 82.

68. Nietzsche, "Uber Wahrheit und Lüge," p. 182 (my translation); "On Truth and Lies," p. 84.

69. Hume, *Enquiry,* ed. Selby-Bigge, p. 112.

70. Friedrich Kessler and Grant Gilmore, *Contracts: Cases and Materials,* 2nd ed. (Boston: Little, Brown, 1970), pp. 3–6.

71. Freud, *Three Essays on the Theory of Sexuality, SE* VII, 144n1 (actually at the bottom of p. 146). And see Arnold I. Davidson, "How to Do the History of Psychoanalysis: A Reading of Freud's *Three Essays on the Theory of Sexuality,*" in Françoise Meltzer, *The Trial(s) of Psychoanalysis* (Chicago and London: University of Chicago Press, 1988), pp. 39–64.

72. Arnold Isenberg, "Deontology and the Ethics of Lying," *Philosophy and Phenomenological Research* 24 (1964): 463–480.

73. Proust, *Remembrance of Things Past,* vol. 1, pp. 390–391.

74. Isaiah Berlin, *Four Essays on Liberty* (Oxford: Clarendon Press, 1968), especially "Two Concepts of Liberty" (1957), pp. 118–138.

75. Alasdair MacIntyre, *After Virtue,* 2nd ed. (London: Duckworth, 1985), pp. 23ff.

76. Karl Marx, *Grundrisse: Foundations of the Critique of Political Economy (Rough Draft),* trans. with foreword by Martin Nicolaus (Harmondsworth: Penguin, 1973), pp. 241–245.

77. Jon Elster, *Sour Grapes: Studies in the Subversion of Rationality* (Cambridge: Cambridge University Press, 1983), p. 155.

78. Herman Melville, *The Confidence-Man* (1857), with an introduction by Tony Tanner (Oxford: Oxford University Press, 1989), p. 295; see Tanner's introduction, esp. pp. xxxiv–xxxvii. See also Leon Howard, *Herman Melville: A Biography* (Berkeley and Los Angeles: University of California Press, 1951), p. 229.

79. See Diego Gambetta, ed., *Trust* (Oxford: Blackwell, 1988).

80. The editor of the *Grundrisse* refers the reader to Aristotle, *Nicomachean Ethics*, book V, chap. 5, para. 14, but I have not been able to find the phrase there; see Aristotle, *Complete Works II*, ed. Jonathan Barnes (Princeton: Princeton University Press, 1984), p. 1788, 1133a7–1133b28.

81. Marx, *Grundrisse*, p. 160.

82. Bob Dylan, "It's Alright Ma," *Bringing It All Back Home* (1965).

83. Walter Bagehot, *Lombard Street: A Description of the Money Market* (London, 1873), p. 68, quoted in S. Herbert Frankel, *Money: Two Philosophies* (Oxford: Basil Blackwell, 1977), p. 31.

84. Dostoevsky's *The Idiot* would serve equally well.

85. Henrik Ibsen, *The Public Enemy*, trans. Peter Watts, in *Ghosts. A Public Enemy. When We Dead Awake* (Harmondsworth: Penguin, 1964), p. 219.

86. Ibid., p. 186. Parentheses in text.

87. Harvey Sacks, "Everyone Has to Lie," in B. G. Blount and Mary Sanches, eds., *Sociocultural Dimensions of Language Use* (New York: Academic Press, 1975), pp. 57–79.

88. Taking the question from J. L. Austin, "Performative Utterances" (1956), in *Philosophical Papers*, 2nd ed., ed. J. O. Urmson and G. J. Warnock (Oxford: Oxford University Press, 1970), p. 249.

89. Think how often battles over whether an insult was "intended" are avoided with the phrase: "I was only joking"; think how many marriages have been saved—or doomed—by the phrase "I was drunk."

90. This is one of the important points that Derrida makes in his "Signature Event Context" and "Limited Inc a b c . . ."; the point is made in large part because we have no way of deciding—nor would "we" (as opposed to "Searle") want to—whether Derrida is joking or not. See "Signature Event Context," *Glyph* 1 (1977): 172–197; "Limited Inc a b c . . .," *Glyph* 2 (1977): 162–254.

91. Thomas Hobbes, *Leviathan* (1651), edited with an introduction by C. B. Macpherson (Harmondsworth: Penguin, 1951), part I, chap. 4, p. 105.

92. The idea that the most important property of a proposition was whether it was true or false was one of the targets of Austin's *How to Do Things with Words;* I am greatly indebted to that seminal work. The fact that such "scientism" was a chief, if not the chief, target of his critique somehow got obscured in many of the later readings.

93. On this see the admirable discussion in Bruno Latour, *Science in Action* (Milton Keynes: Open University Press, 1987), esp. pp. 1–100.

94. For a survey of the ancient sources and discussion on the Cretan Liar Paradox, see Alexander Rüstow, *Der Lügner: Theorie/Geschichte und Auflösung*, Inaugural Dissertation, Erlangen, 1908 (Leipzig: Teubner, 1910); for a comprehensive list of textual sources, see pp. 142–145.

95. R. M. Sainsbury, *Paradoxes* (Cambridge: Cambridge University Press), p. 1.

96. Ibid.

97. Bertrand Russell, *Autobiography: 1872–1914* (London: George Allen and Unwin, 1967), p. 147.

98. Ludwig Wittgenstein, *Remarks on the Foundations of Mathematics*, 3rd ed., ed. G. H. von Wright, R. Rhees, and G. E. M. Anscombe, trans. G. E. M. Anscombe (Oxford: Blackwell, 1978), p. 207.

99. In what follows, I rely heavily upon the admirably lucid discussion in Sainsbury, *Paradoxes*, chapter 5.

100. Frank P. Ramsey, "The Foundations of Mathematics" (1925), reprinted in D. H. Mellor, ed., *Foundations* (Atlantic Highlands, N.J.: Humanities Press, 1978), pp. 171–172.

101. Alfred Tarski, "The Concept of Truth in Formalized Languages," in Tarski, *Logic, Semantics, Metamathematics* (New York: Clarendon Press, 1956), pp. 152–278.

102. James Cargile, *Paradoxes* (Cambridge: Cambridge University Press, 1979).

103. Karl Popper, "Self Reference and Meaning in Ordinary Language," in Popper, *Conjectures and Refutations*, 3rd ed. (London: Routledge and Kegan Paul, 1969), pp.304–311; this passage from p. 310.

104. Sainsbury, *Paradoxes*, p. 122.

105. In particular, we see clearly that, as Sainsbury points out, truth requires some "grounding," and statements such as "This statement is false" and "This statement is true" are insufficiently grounded. This problem is that of language: language is derivative of the world, and not vice versa. We would think it odd if there were only language in the world, but do not have much problem imagining a world without language. We therefore assume that language is derivative of the world. Yet all natural languages go beyond this function and exceed their proper relation to the world. We have only to think of Augustine's proof of the existence of God through the eternal nature of truth to see that Platonism lends itself readily to a view of language (the Forms) as somehow deeper and more enduring than the world. To put the point bluntly if not altogether accurately, the paradoxes remind us of the continual temptation, inherent in our language(s), to make language (or truth, or ideas) more than the world. The Nietzschean antidote to these idealisms is to assert, paradoxically, that the lie precedes truth.

106. Alfred Tarski, "Truth and Proof," *Scientific American* 220, no. 6 (June 1969): 63–77.

107. James Cargile, "Paradoxes," in *The Oxford Companion to Philosophy,*

ed. Ted Honderich (Oxford and New York: Oxford University Press, 1995), p. 644.

108. Lewis Carroll, "What the Tortoise Said to Achilles" (1895), reprinted in Douglas Hofstadter, *Gödel, Escher, Bach* (1979) (Harmondsworth: Penguin, 1980), pp. 43–45.

109. Gregory Bateson, *Steps towards an Ecology of Mind* (London: Paladin, 1973), pp. 173–198.

110. Wittgenstein, *Remarks on the Foundations of Mathematics,* p. 255.

111. Ludwig Wittgenstein, *Philosophical Investigations,* 3rd ed. (Oxford: Basil Blackwell, 1967), para. 249; see also para. 668 and p. 222.

112. Jacques Lacan, *The Four Fundamental Concepts of Psychoanalysis* (Seminar XI, 1963–1964), trans. Alan Sheridan (London: Tavistock, 1977), p. 140; see also pp. 233–234.

113. Freud, *Jokes and Their Relation to the Unconscious, SE* VIII, 115.

114. Ibid.

115. Similar incorporations of the position of the other have emerged in developments in analytic philosophy associated with speech act theory and Grice's maxims concerning the charity conditions governing communication; see the discussion of the maxim "Make your contribution as uninformative (weak) as is compatible with the purpose of the discourse" in Jaakko Hintikka, "Logic of Conversation as a Logic of Dialogue," in Richard E. Grandy and Richard Warner, eds., *Philosophical Grounds of Rationality: Intentions, Categories, Ends* (Oxford: Clarendon Press, 1986), pp. 259–276, esp. p. 270, and the primacy of utterer's meaning over "the abstract concept of literal meaning" in Patrick Suppes, "The Primacy of Utterer's Meaning," in Grandy and Warner, *Philosophical Grounds of Rationality,* pp. 109–129, esp. p. 113.

116. Harry Frankfurt, "On Bullshit," *Raritan Review* 6 (1986): 81–100; this passage from p. 94.

117. John von Neumann and Oscar Morgenstern, *The Theory of Games and Economic Behavior* (Princeton, N.J.: Princeton University Press, 1944); see E. Roy Weintraub, ed., *Toward a History of Game Theory* (Durham and London: Duke University Press, 1992).

118. See Lloyd Gerson, "Augustine's Neoplatonic Argument for the Existence of God," *The Thomist* 45 (1981): 571–584, and the discussion in Peter Dear, "Mersenne and the Learning of the Schools: Continuity and Transformation in the Scientific Revolution" (Ph.D. dissertation, Princeton University, 1984), p. 147 and n. 89.

119. Nicolaas A. Rupke, *The Great Chain of History: William Buckland and the English School of Geology (1814–1849)* (Oxford: Clarendon Press, 1983).

120. Norbert Wiener, *The Human Use of Human Beings* (1950) (London: Sphere, 1968), p. 34.

121. Ibid., pp. 34–35; see also Peter Galison, "The Ontology of the Enemy: Norbert Wiener and the Cybernetic Vision," *Critical Inquiry* 21 (1994).

122. Steven Shapin, *A Social History of Truth: Civility and Science in Seventeenth-Century England* (Chicago: University of Chicago Press, 1994), p. 417.

123. Alfred C. Haddon, *History of Anthropology* (London: Watts, 1910), pp. 85–86.

124. Herbert C. Kelman, "Behavioral Research," in *Encyclopaedia of Bioethics*, ed. Warren T. Reich (London: Collier Macmillan/Free Press, 1978), vol. 4, pp. 1470–1481.

125. Stanley Milgram, "Some Conditions of Obedience and Disobedience to Authority," *Human Relations* 18 (1965): 57–75; Milgram, *Obedience to Authority* (New York: Harper and Row, 1974); for details of the experiments see Appendix I, pp. 193–202.

126. Milgram, *Obedience to Authority*, p. 128.

127. Margaret Mead, "Research with Human Beings: A Model Derived from Anthropological Field Practice," *Daedalus* 98, no. 2 (1969): 361–386; this passage from p. 375.

128. For a good survey of both the history and the issues involved, see Ruth R. Faden and Tom L. Beauchamp in collaboration with Nancy M. P. King, *A History and Theory of Informed Consent* (New York and Oxford: Oxford University Press, 1986), esp. pp. 167ff.

129. The translation in Immanuel Kant, *Critique of Pure Reason*, trans. Norman Kemp Smith (London: Macmillan, 1933), p. 20 reads: "reason has insight only into that which it produces after a plan of its own, and that it must not allow itself to be kept, as it were, in nature's leading-strings, but must itself show the way with principles of judgment based upon fixed laws, constraining nature to give answer to questions of reason's own determining." I follow Gay's translation in Peter Gay, *The Enlightenment: An Interpretation*, 2 vols. (London: Weidenfeld and Nicolson, 1969), vol. 2, p. 8.

130. Mead, "Research with Human Beings," p. 375n.

131. Laud Humphreys, *Tearoom Trade: Impersonal Sex in Public Places* (London: Duckworth, 1974), "Postscript: A Question of Ethics," p. 168.

132. Harold Garfinkel, "A Conception of, and Experiments with 'Trust' as a Condition of Stable Concerted Actions," in O. J. Harvey, ed., *Motivation and Social Interaction* (New York: Ronald Press, 1963), pp. 187–238; Harold Garfinkel, *Studies in Ethnomethodology* (Englewood Cliffs, N.J.: Prentice-Hall,

1967); Michael Lynch, *Scientific Practice and Ordinary Action: Ethnomethodology and Social Studies of Science* (Cambridge: Cambridge University Press, 1993).

133. H. M. Collins, "The Meaning of Lies: Accounts of Action and Participatory Research," in *Accounts and Action*, ed. G. Nigel Gilbert and Peter Abell, Surrey Conference on Sociological Theory and Method, vol. 1. (Aldershot: Gower, 1983), pp. 69–76; this passage from pp. 71–72. See also Augustine Brannigan and Michael Lynch, "On Bearing False Witness: Credibility as an Interactional Accomplishment," *Journal of Contemporary Ethnography* 16 (1987): 115–146.

134. See Stephen A. Ambrose, *Duty, Honor, Country: A History of West Point* (Baltimore: Johns Hopkins University Press, 1966), p. 51, discussed in John Tresch, "Engineering the Artificial Paradise: The Facts in the Case of Edgar A. Poe," M.Phil. dissertation, Department of History and Philosophy of Science, Cambridge University, June 1996.

135. J. D. Frank, *Persuasion and Healing* (New York: Schocken, 1963).

136. L. J. Henderson, "Physician and Patient as a Social System," *New England Journal of Medicine* 212 (1935): 819–823, quoted in Tom L. Beauchamp and James F. Childress, *Principles of Biomedical Ethics*, 4th ed. (New York and Oxford: Oxford University Press, 1994), p. 276.

137. Beauchamp and Childress, *Principles*, p. 398.

138. Milan Kundera, *Immortality*, trans. Peter Kussi (London and Boston: Faber and Faber, 1991), pp. 122–124.

139. Bok, *Lying*, p. 66, and Howard Spiro, *Doctors, Patients, and Placebos* (New Haven: Yale University Press, 1986), p. 27.

140. H. Brody, "The Lie that Heals: The Ethics of Giving Placebos," *Annals of Internal Medicine* 97 (1982): 112–118.

141. W. R. Houston, "The Doctor Himself as a Therapeutic Agent," *Annals of Internal Medicine* 11 (1938): 1416–1425.

142. Spiro, *Doctors, Patients, and Placebos*, p. 23.

143. Ibid., p. 44. The figures that follow are mainly drawn from Spiro's survey.

144. L. A. Cobb, C. F. Kittle, and J. E. Crockett, "An Evaluation of Internal Mammary Artery Ligation by a Double Blind Technique," *New England Journal of Medicine* 260 (1959): 1115–1118; E. G. Dimond, C. F. Kittle and J. E. Crockett, "Comparison of Internal Mammary Artery Ligation and Sham Operation for Angina Pectoris," *American Journal of Cardiology* 5 (1960): 483–486.

145. M. Vlades et al., "'Sham Operations' Revisited: A Comparison of Complete vs. Unsuccessful Coronary Artery Bypass," *American Journal of Cardiology* 43 (1979): 382; see Daniel E. Moerman, "Physiology and Symbols: The

Anthropological Implications of the Placebo Effect," in L. Romancieci-Ross, D. E. Moerman, and L. R. Tancredi, eds., *The Anthropology of Medicine* (New York: Praeger, 1983), pp. 156–167.

146. Alan H. Roberts, Donald G. Kewman, Lisa Mercier, and Mel Hovell, "The Power of Nonspecific Effects in Healing: Implications for Psychosocial and Biological Treatments," *Clinical Psychology Review* 13 (1993): 375–391.

147. Spiro, *Doctors, Patients, and Placebos*, p. 91.

148. See ibid., p. 30, for these figures and sources.

149. Ibid., p. 86.

150. See Beauchamp and Childress, *Principles*, pp. 442ff.

151. Spiro, *Doctors, Patients, and Placebos*, p. 44.

152. Ibid., p. 12.

153. Ibid., p. 16.

154. Bok, *Lying*, p. 63.

155. Interview with Marcel Colin, "La clinique criminologique, une approche pluridisciplinaire," *Nervures* 7 (October 1988), cited in Daniel Zagury, "La clinique psychiatrique n'est plus ce qu'elle était . . .," *Nouvelle Revue de Psychanalyse* 42 (Fall 1990): 121–135, this quote from p. 131: "Outside of the will to cure, there is no scientific knowledge in medicine. Within the framework of our epistemology, deprived of therapeutic commitment, the simple diagnostic exercise, the pure gaze is worth nothing."

## II: Lying on the Couch

1. Thomas Sydenham, *Epistolary Dissertation*, in *The Entire Works of Dr. Thomas Sydenham* (London: Cave, 1753), quoted in E. M. Thornton, *Hypnotism, Hysteria, and Epilepsy: An Historical Synthesis* (London: Heinemann, 1975), p. 123.

2. Jules Falret, "Folie raisonnante ou folie morale" (speech presented to the Société Médico-psychologique, 8 January 1866), in *Etudes cliniques sur les maladies mentales et nerveuses* (Paris: Baillière, 1890), p. 502, quoted in Jacques Lagrange, "Versions de la psychanalyse dans le texte de Foucault," *Psychanalyse à l'Université* 12 (1987): 261n9.

3. J. M. Masson, *Against Therapy. Warning: Psychotherapy May Be Hazardous to Your Mental Health* (London: Collins, 1989), pp. 49–83.

4. See Carl Gustav Jung and Frederick Peterson, "Psychophysical Investigations with the Galvonometer and Pneumograph in Normal and Insane Individuals" (1907), in Jung, *Collected Works*, vol. 2, *Experimental Researches*, trans. Leopold Stein in collaboration with Diana Riviere (London: Routledge

and Kegan Paul, 1973), pp. 492–553; Paul Ekman, *Telling Lies: Clues to Deceit in the Marketplace, Politics, and Marriage* (New York: Norton, 1985); Anthony Gale, ed., *The Polygraph Test: Lies, Truth, and Science* (London: Sage, 1988); D. T. Lykken, *A Tremor in the Blood: Uses and Abuses of the Lie Detector* (New York and London: McGraw-Hill, 1981).

5. On the possibility of the Frye Standard being superseded by the consequences of the *Daubert vs. Merrill Dow* ruling of 1993 in the U.S. Supreme Court (introducing a key new element of scientificity, namely the principle or discovery having been subjected to peer review), see Sheila Jasanoff, "A Higher Law: The U.S. Supreme Court and the Reliability of Science," paper presented to the Cambridge Group for the History of Psychiatry, Psychoanalysis, and Allied Sciences Seminar, 15 May 1996.

6. *Frye v. U.S.*, 293 F. 1013 (D.C.Cir. 1923), also cited in Steven Emanuel, *Evidence*, second edition with the assistance of Renée Samuelson (Larchmont, N.Y.: Emanuel Law Outlines, 1991). p. 414. Note that other scientific evidence has bypassed the Frye Standard, and, especially in the recent past, has been accepted by courts without evidence of its "general acceptance," for example, neutron activation analysis.

7. Bruno Latour, *Les Microbes, Guerre et Paix, suivi de Irréductions* (Paris: Anne-Marie Métailié, 1984), p. 253; my translation.

8. How what became known as the "behavioral sciences" went about constructing the ideal (and also the excluded) subject of their experiments is beyond the scope of this essay. It is clearly of great importance. For instance, in the Würzburg School's famous experiments, Professor Külpe was himself the person under examination in the experiments (as also was clearly true in "introspective" experiments, such as Francis Galton's "discovery" of free association in the late 1870s). By the 1930s the "observer," as he had been called by the Würzburg school, had become a "subject" who must not know what the experiment is about, could therefore never participate in an experiment twice, and should possess little or no "learning," particularly in the field being ploughed by the experimenters. See Kurt Danziger, *Constructing the Subject: Historical Origins of Psychological Research* (Cambridge: Cambridge University Press, 1990), and on the Würzburgers, Martin Kusch, "Recluse, Interlocutor, Interrogator: Natural and Social Order in Turn-of-the-Century Psychological Research Schools," *Isis* 86 (1995): 419–439, and Adrian C. Brock, "Imageless Thought or Stimulus Error? The Social Construction of Psychological Expertise," in William R. Woodward and Robert S. Cohen, eds., *World Views and Scientific Discipline Formation* (Dordrecht: Kluwer, 1991), pp. 97–106.

9. Jeffrey M. Masson, *The Assault on Truth: Freud's Suppression of the*

*Seduction Theory* (London: Faber and Faber, 1984); see also Ann Scott, *Real Events Revisited: Fantasy, Memory, and Psychoanalysis* (London: Virago, 1996).

10. Jacques Lacan, *The Seminar. Book I. Freud's Papers on Technique. 1953–54*, ed. Jacques-Alain Miller, trans. with notes by John Forrester (Cambridge: Cambridge University Press, 1988), pp. 174–175.

11. *ID, SE* V, 515–516: "There is in general no guarantee of the correctness of our memory; and yet we yield to the compulsion to attach belief to its data far more often than is objectively justified . . . in analyzing a dream I insist that the whole scale of estimates of certainty shall be abandoned and that the faintest possibility that something of this or that sort may have occurred in the dream shall be treated as absolute certainty."

12. Freud, "Negation," *SE* XIX, 235; *Stud* III, 373.

13. *ID, SE* V, 461–462; translation modified.

14. *FF*, 21 September 1897, p. 264. This is the third of the reasons Freud gave in the autumn of 1897 for discarding the seduction theory.

15. "If I were depressed, confused, exhausted, such doubts would surely have to be interpreted as signs of weakness. Since I am in an opposite state, I must recognize them as the result of honest and vigorous intellectual work and must be proud that after going so deep I am still capable of such criticism. Can it be that this doubt merely represents an episode in the advance toward further insight?" *FF*, 21 September 1897, p. 265. Note the analytic attitude Freud adopts towards his own "doubt."

16. Freud, "Hypnotism," *SE* I, 110. Strachey adds an acute footnote, drawing the reader's attention to the "agreement with the ego" (*SE* XXIII, 239) upon which psychoanalysis is based.

17. Freud, "Hypnotism," *SE* I, 113.

18. Ibid. On the relation of the "playing a part" in psychoanalytic treatment to the transference, it would be suggestive to compare these remarks with Freud's comments at the end of the "Dora" case history.

19. Jean-Luc Donnet, "Le devenir d'une scène de séduction," *Études Freudiennes*, no. 27 (March 1986): 49.

20. Freud, in Herman Nunberg and Ernst Federn, eds., *Minutes of the Vienna Psychoanalytical Society, Vol. III: 1910–1911* (New York: International Universities Press, 1974), 19 October 1910, p. 23.

21. See Norman Malcolm, *Dreaming* (London: Routledge and Kegan Paul, 1959).

22. Elmer Lee, "How Far Does a Scientific Therapy Depend upon the Materia Medica in the Cure of Disease?" *Journal of the American Medical Association* 31 (8 October 1898): 827, quoted in Charles Rosenberg, "The Thera-

peutic Revolution: Medicine, Meaning, and Social Change in Nineteenth-century America" in Morris J. Vogel and Charles E. Rosenberg, eds., *The Therapeutic Revolution: Essays in the Social History of American Medicine* (Philadelphia: University of Pennsylvania Press, 1979), pp. 3–25; this quote from p. 19.

23. Freud, "Psychical Treatment" (1890), *SE* VII, 298.

24. Freud, "Explanations, Applications, and Orientations," *New Introductory Lectures*, *SE* XXII, 152.

25. Freud, "Studies on Hysteria," *SE* II, 304.

26. John Forrester, "The Balance of Power between Freud and His Early Women Patients," in André Haynal and Ernst Falzeder, eds., *100 Years of Psychoanalysis: Contributions to the History of Psychoanalysis, Cahiers Psychiatriques Genevois, Special Issue* (Geneva: Institutions Universitaires de Psychiatrie de Genève, Psychiatriques, 1994), pp. 41–54.

27. The German phrase translated by Strachey as "indications of reality" is *Realitätszeichen*—signs or markers of reality.

28. Saying that it is an artifice of the analytic situation does not mean that it is explicitly excluded that one can observe it outside that situation; but these observations do not count for very much, in the same way that "observations" of electrons outside the laboratory, the electricity grid, the telescope, and the computer do not count for very much.

29. Calls by psychoanalysts on their colleagues to recognize the "reality" of the analyst—in particular, his or her personal response to the patient, to the events of the analysis, and so forth—do not, in my opinion, fundamentally change this primitive datum. The analyst is bound to *conceal* much of his private life, inner thoughts, and so forth—for "technical" reasons: that is, for purposes to do solely (or overwhelmingly) with the conduct of the conversation.

30. This analogy is suggested by the brilliant discussion of the jealous lover as scientist in Malcolm Bowie, *Freud, Proust, and Lacan: Theory as Fiction* (Cambridge: Cambridge University Press, 1987), esp. p. 55.

31. See my "Contracting the Disease of Love" on the way in which analysis puts all discourses in question, and my "Rape, Seduction, and Psychoanalysis" for the specific immiscibility of legal and psychoanalytic discourse, both in Forrester, *The Seductions of Psychoanalysis*. Leslie Farber, "Lying on the Couch," *Review of Existential Psychology and Psychiatry* 13, no. 2 (1974): 125–135, argues that the dramatic revelations of the unconscious to which the technique of free association lends itself are a form of lying, the form of lying specific to and encouraged by psychoanalysis. His formulation of the argument, also found in Lacan, concerning the paradoxical relation of psychoanalysis to the truth, is exemplary: "The entire enterprise of psychoanalysis is predicated on a person's

capacity for truth-telling. And yet the very devices and strategies traditionally employed for facilitating his search for truth (devised . . . to outwit his *in*capacity for truth-telling) not to mention the tools for deciphering and celebrating the truth, once it is found—all seem to encourage the patient's capacity to embellish, to dramatize,—in short, to lie" (p. 131). This important recognition is tantamount to conceding that there is never any guarantee, either at the beginning or the end of the process of truth-seeking, that one can distinguish fiction from truth. All the more reason, one might conclude, to adopt the singular epistemology that psychoanalysis embodies.

32. Trilling, *Freud and the Crisis of Our Culture* (Boston: Beacon Press, 1955), p. 20.

33. Michael Balint, *The Basic Fault: Therapeutic Aspects of Regression* (London: Tavistock, 1968), p. 167.

34. Freud, "Analysis of a Phobia in a Five Year Old Boy" (1909), *SE* X, 129.

35. Ibid., pp. 102–103.

36. Freud, "Two Lies Told by Children," *SE* XII, 305.

37. Ibid., p. 308.

38. Ibid., pp. 308–309.

39. The identity of this patient has now been deduced; she has been shown to be the subject of a number of other important papers of Freud's in this period, as well as being much discussed in his correspondence with Jung and with Pfister. See Ernst Falzeder, "My Grand-Patient, My Chief Tormentor: A Hitherto Unnoticed Case of Freud's and the Consequences," *Psychoanalytic Quarterly* 63 (1994): 297–331.

40. Freud, "Two Lies Told by Children," *SE* XII, 305.

41. Ibid., p. 306.

42. Ibid., p. 307.

43. Ibid., p. 306.

44. Ibid., p. 309; *Stud* V, 234.

45. "Thoughts for the Time on War and Death," *SE* XIV, 276.

46. Ibid., p. 279.

47. Freud, *The Future of an Illusion, SE* XXI, 12.

48. Helene Deutsch, "On the Pathological Lie (pseudologia fantastica)" (1922), *Journal of the American Academy of Psychoanalysis* 10 (1982): 369–386; Friedrich-Wilhelm Eickhoff, "Versuch über die Lüge aus psychoanalytischer Sicht," *Jahrbuch der Psychoanalyse* 23 (1988): 82–101; Otto Fenichel, "The Economics of Pseudologia Fantastica," in *Collected Papers, Second Series* (New York: Norton, 1954), pp. 129–140; Robert Langs, "Truth Therapy, Lie Therapy," *International Journal of Psychoanalysis and Psychotherapy* 8 (1980–1981):

3–34; Edna O'Shaugnessy, "Can a Liar Be Psychoanalysed?" *International Journal of Psycho-Analysis* 71 (1990): 187–195.

49. Sándor Ferenczi, "The Principle of Relaxation and Neocatharsis" (1929), in Ferenczi, *Final Contributions to the Problems and Methods of Psycho-analysis,* ed. Michael Balint, trans. Eric Mosbacher et al. (London: Hogarth Press and the Institute of Psycho-analysis, 1955), pp. 108–125; this quote from pp. 120–121.

50. Ibid., p. 121.

51. Ferenczi, "The Problem of the Termination of the Analysis," in Ferenczi, *Final Contributions,* pp. 77–86; this passage from p. 77.

52. Ibid., p. 78.

53. Ibid., p. 77.

54. Ibid., p. 78.

55. Freud, "Negation," *SE* XIX, 239.

56. Wittgenstein, *Philosophical Investigations,* no. 447, p. 131e.

57. Laurence R. Horn, *A Natural History of Negation* (Chicago and London: University of Chicago Press, 1989), p. 203.

58. Ferenczi, "Termination," p. 79.

59. Ibid., p. 81.

60. Ibid., p. 83.

61. Ferenczi, "The Principle of Relaxation and Neocatharsis," p. 115.

62. Ibid., p. 117.

63. Adam Phillips, *Terrors and Experts* (London and Boston: Faber and Faber/Harvard University Press, 1995), p. 6; see John Forrester, "Casualties of Truth," chapter 2 in Forrester, *Dispatches from the Freud Wars* (Cambridge, Mass.: Harvard University Press, 1997), pp. 44–106.

64. Freud, "Observations on Transference-love," *SE* XIV, 164.

65. See Lisa Appignanesi and John Forrester, *Freud's Women* (London: Weidenfeld and Nicolson; New York: Basic Books, 1992), p. 214.

66. A critical Freud scholar might point to Freud's discussion of the lying dreams and deceptive actions of the female homosexual whose case history he published in 1920 (*SE* XVIII, 147–172) as evidence of his being decidedly ruffled by the latent hostility concealed behind, and revealed by, the patient's mendacity, to the point where he broke off the treatment and passed her to another analyst. That this reading is superficial is shown by the discussion in Appignanesi and Forrester, *Freud's Women,* pp. 182–189, which argues in detail that, like the patient's mother, but in contrast to her father, neither the patient's homosexuality nor her lies and hypocrisy troubled Freud. It is also clear from Freud's tone that he takes some pleasure in catching out those analysts like

Ferenczi who "idealize" the unconscious as the seat of all psychic truth by putting the views quoted in the epigraph to this section in their mouths.

67. Edna O'Shaugnessy, "Can a Liar Be Psychoanalysed?" p. 194.

68. Freud, "The Psychogenesis of a Case of Homosexuality in a Woman" (1920), *SE* XVIII, 164.

69. A point recognized by Farber in his elegant and thoughtful paper "Lying on the Couch," part of a special issue of the journal *Review of Existential Psychology and Psychiatry* devoted to lying (vol. 13, no. 2, 1974), with notable contributions by Leo Kovar, Robert Boyers, and Joyce Carol Oates.

70. Freud, *An Autobiographical Study*, *SE* XX, 30.

71. Freud, "Dreams and Telepathy," *SE* XVIII, 204.

72. See Amélie Oksenberg Rorty, "The Deceptive Self: Liars, Layers, and Lairs," in *Perspectives on Self-deception*, ed. Brian P. McLaughlin and Amélie Oksenberg Rorty (Berkeley: University of California Press, 1988), pp. 11–28; Donald Davidson, "Paradoxes of Irrationality," in James Hopkins and Richard Wollheim, eds., *Philosophical Essays on Freud* (Cambridge: Cambridge University Press, 1984), pp. 289–305; Donald Davidson, "Deception and Division," in *Actions and Events*, ed. E. LePore and B. McLaughlin (New York: Basil Blackwell, 1985); Elster, *Sour Grapes*, esp. p. 149. The most penetrating overall analysis of self-deception in relation to psychoanalysis is Sebastian Gardner, *Irrationality and the Philosophy of Psychoanalysis* (Cambridge: Cambridge University Press, 1993).

73. Sartre, *Being and Nothingness*, p. 92.

74. Sándor Ferenczi, "To Whom Does One Relate One's Dreams?" in *Further Contributions to the Theory and Technique of Psycho-analysis*, compiled by John Rickman, trans. Jane Isabel Suttie et al. (London: The Hogarth Press and Institute of Psycho-analysis, 1926), p. 349.

75. Lacan, *The Seminar. Book II. The Ego in Freud's Theory and in the Technique of Psychoanalysis*, ed. Jacques-Alain Miller, trans. Sylvana Tomaselli, with notes by John Forrester (Cambridge: Cambridge University Press; New York: Norton, 1988), pp. 262ff.

76. In *Le Séminaire. Livre VI. Le Désir et son Interprétation. 1958–1959;* see J.-B. Pontalis, "Comptes Rendu," *Bulletin de Psychologie* 13 (1959–1960): 269–270.

77. *E* 251–252/43, "Fonction et champ de la parole et du langage en psychanalyse"; translation modified.

78. Christopher Bollas, *The Shadow of the Object: Psychoanalysis and the Thought Unknown* (London: Free Association Books, 1987), p. 185.

79. Ibid.

80. Ibid., p. 186.

81. From a huge literature, I select Ian Hacking, *Rewriting the Soul: Multiple Personality and the Sciences of Memory* (Princeton, N.J.: Princeton University Press, 1995).

82. R. D. Laing, *Wisdom, Madness, and Folly: The Making of a Psychiatrist, 1927–1957* (London: Macmillan, 1985), pp. 126–128.

83. The issues raised by requirements to report the content of analytic sessions to the police are examined in a brilliantly clear and strong-minded fashion in Christopher Bollas and David Sundelson, *The New Informants: The Betrayal of Confidentiality in Psychoanalysis and Psychotherapy* (New York: Jason Aronson; London: Karnac, 1995). The fact of Bollas's interest in the issues involved in reporting the confidential communications of a patient to an outside authority gives an added twist to his lying patient's maneuvers concerning his intended murder.

84. Justice Tobriner, Majority Opinion, *Tarasoff v. Regents of the University of California*, 17 Cal.3d 425 (1976); 131 *California Reporter* 14 (1 July 1976), partially excerpted in Beauchamp and Childress, *Principles of Biomedical Ethics*, Appendix, "Cases in Biomedical Ethics," p. 511.

85. Beauchamp and Childress, *Principles of Biomedical Ethics*, p. 425.

86. Justice Clark, Dissenting Opinion, *Tarasoff v. Regents of the University of California*, in Beauchamp and Childress, *Principles of Biomedical Ethics*, p. 512.

87. Freud, "Psycho-analysis and the Establishment of the Facts in Legal Proceedings" (1906), *SE* IX, 113.

88. Carol Gilligan, "Recovering Psyche: A Psychology of Love and a Politics of Resistance," paper presented to the Cambridge Group for the History of Psychiatry, Psychoanalysis, and Allied Sciences, 3 March 1993.

89. Friedrich Nietzsche, *The Gay Science* (1887), trans. with commentary by Walter Kaufmann (New York: Random House, 1974), para. 344, p. 281.

90. Ibid., pp. 282–283.

## Gift, Money, and Debt

1. There are moments, however, in the *Ecrits* where there is a flurry of page references to Freud's text (for example, "Intervention sur le transfert"); but even when he is closely following a text, and directing his reader's attention to that text, Lacan does not quote it directly.

2. *E* 435/144.

3. *E* 142 (Engl.), "The Freudian Thing."

4. The French version of this text that I have used, in much the same spirit that one listens to *Leonore 2* rather than *3*, is the unpublished 1953 version issued by the Centre de la Documentation Universitaire, a copy of which was deposited in the Bibliothèque Nationale, Paris. A very similar version was published in *Ornicar?* in 1978. I will also give page references to the English translation by Martha Noel Evans, "The Neurotic's Individual Myth," *Psychoanalytic Quarterly* 48 (1979): 405–425. Hereafter citations will be abbreviated as *Myth*, followed by two page references, the first to the French.

5. *Myth* 6/408; emphasis added, translation modified.

6. *E* 199 (Engl.), "Possible Treatment."

7. *E* 77 (Engl.), "Function and Field."

8. *E* 79 (Engl.), "Function and Field."

9. Freud, "Original Record of the Case," *SE* X, 300; Freud to the Rat Man, 21 December 1907. Note that this volume of the *Standard Edition*, which was the first publication of the Rat Man's case notes, was first published in 1956, some time after most of Lacan's discussions of the Rat Man; hence the original case notes were not available to him. Hereafter, references to these published case notes will be referred to as "Original record."

10. *Myth* 12–13/413.

11. Freud, "Notes upon a Case of Obsessional Neurosis" (hereafter abbreviated as Rat Man), *SE* X, 195–199.

12. "Original record," *SE* X, 293.

13. Ibid., p. 292.

14. Rat Man, *SE* X, 210–211.

15. Ibid.

16. *Myth* 14/414.

17. "Original record," *SE* X, 290.

18. *Myth* 28/425.

19. Ibid., 9/411.

20. Ibid., 18/417.

21. Ibid., 15/415.

22. *E* 302/89, "Function and Field."

23. Rat Man, *SE* X, 182.

24. *E* 353–355, "Variantes de la cure-type."

25. Rat Man, *SE* X, 201.

26. Ibid., p. 166.

27. *E* 290–291, "Function and Field."

28. *Myth* 3–4/407.

29. Ibid., 4/407.

30. Ibid., 4/407–408.

31. Ibid., 25/422.

32. Ibid., 27/423.

33. Lacan, "La Famille," *Encyclopédie Française* (1938), vol. 8, "La Vie Mentale," 8.40, p. 16.

34. Phrase in English in the original.

35. Lacan, "La Famille," 8.40, p. 16.

36. Ibid., 8.42, p. 5.

37. Ibid., 8.42, pp. 6–7.

38. Lacan, "Discussion," *Revue Française de Psychanalyse Comptes Rendus* (April–June 1949): 317.

39. *E* 133, "Introduction Théorique aux Fonctions de la Psychanalyse en Criminologie" (1950).

40. Lacan, *Seminaire IX. L'identification* (1961–1962), Session 16, p. 9 (unpublished).

41. *E* 143 (Engl.), "The Freudian Thing."

42. *E* 278/67, "Fonction et champ."

43. Rat Man, *SE* X, 173.

44. *Myth* 13/414.

45. Rat Man, *SE* X, 172.

46. *E* 302, "Fonction et champ."

47. *E* 354–355, "Variantes de la cure-type."

48. See Freud, "Screen Memories," *SE* III, 314; William J. McGrath, *Freud's Discovery of Psychoanalysis: The Politics of Hysteria* (Ithaca and London: Cornell University Press, 1986), pp. 129–131; Peter J. Swales, "Freud, Martha Bernays and the Language of Flowers, Masturbation, Cocaine, and the Inflation of Fantasy," privately printed, 1983, esp. pp. 33–37; Lisa Appignanesi and John Forrester, *Freud's Women* (London: Weidenfeld and Nicolson/New York: Basic, 1992), pp. 22–25.

49. See Freud, "On Dreams," *SE* V, 636–639, and Didier Anzieu, *L'Autoanalyse de Freud* (Paris: Presses Universitaires de France, 1975).

50. *E* 143 (Engl.), "The Freudian Thing." See John P. Muller and William J. Richardson, *Lacan and Language: A Reader's Guide to Ecrits* (New York: International Universities Press, 1982), p. 159, for a correction of the translation of this passage.

51. *ID, SE* IV, 216.

52. Rat Man, *SE* X, 205.

53. *ID, SE* IV, 205.

54. A version of the Shakespearian "thou owest God a death."

55. *E* 143 (Engl.), "The Freudian Thing."

56. *E* 199 (Engl.), "Possible Treatment."

57. *E* 251–252, "Fonction et champ."

58. Lacan, *Le Séminaire. Livre I. Les Écrits Techniques de Freud. 1953–1954* (Paris: Seuil, 1975); *The Seminar. Book I. Freud's Papers on Technique 1953–1954*, trans. with notes by John Forrester (Cambridge: Cambridge University Press/New York: Norton, 1988), p. 157.

59. Stéphane Mallarmé, *The Poems*, trans. and introduction by Keith Bosley (Harmondsworth: Penguin, 19XX), pp. 44–47: "Narrer, enseigner, même décrire, cela va et encore qu'à chacun suffirait peut-être pour échanger la pensée humaine, de prendre ou de mettre dans la main d'autrui en silence une pièce de monnaie, l'emploi élémentaire du discours dessert l'universel *reportage* dont, la littérature exceptée, participe tout entre les genres d'écrits contemporains" (translation modified).

60. Freud, *Studies on Hysteria*, *SE* II, 69.

61. Friedrich Nietzsche, *Das Philosophenbuch* (1873), part III, "Knowledge-theoretical Introduction on Truth and Lies in an Extra-moral Sense" (Paris: Aubier Flammarion Bilingue, 1969), p. 182 (my translation); see the English translation in Nietzsche, *Philosophy and Truth: Selections from Nietzsche's Notebooks of the early 1870s*, trans. and edited with an introduction and notes by Daniel Breazeale (Atlantic Highlands, N.J.: Humanities/Hassocks, Sussex: Harvester, 1979), p. 84.

62. *E* 50 (Engl.).

63. Lacan, *Seminar I*, pp. 189–191 (Engl.).

64. Shoshana Felman, *Le Scandale du Corps Parlant* (Paris: Seuil, 1980).

65. Jean Bellemin-Noël, "Psychanalyse et pragmatique," *Critique* 420 (May 1982): 406–422.

66. Mikkel Borch-Jacobsen, *Lacan: Le Maître Absolu* (Paris: Flammarion, 1990); *Lacan: The Absolute Master*, trans. Douglas Brick (Stanford, Calif.: Stanford University Press, 1991).

67. John Forrester, "What the Psychoanalyst Does with Words: Austin, Lacan, and the Speech Acts of Psychoanalysis," in Forrester, *The Seductions of Psychoanalysis: Freud, Lacan, and Derrida* (Cambridge: Cambridge University Press, 1990), pp. 141–167.

68. Jacques Lacan, *The Seminar. Book II. The Ego in Freud's Theory and in the Technique of Psychoanalysis, 1954–1955* (1978), trans. Sylvana Tomaselli, with notes by John Forrester (Cambridge: Cambridge University Press/New York: Norton, 1988), p. 261.

69. *E* 68 (Engl.).

70. *E* 322/106, "Function and Field."

71. *E* 61–62, (Engl.), "Function and Field."

72. Ibid.

73. See Stephen G. Brush, ed., *Kinetic Theory, Vol. II, Irreversible Processes* (Oxford: Pergamon, 1965); Ilya Prigogine and Isabelle Stengers, *Order out of Chaos* (London: Heinemann, 1984).

74. Greg Myers, "Nineteenth-century Popularizations of Thermodynamics and the Rhetoric of Social Prophecy," in Patrick Brantlinger, ed., *Energy and Entropy: Science and Culture in Victorian Britain, Essays from Victorian Studies* (Bloomington and Indianapolis: Indiana University Press, 1989), pp. 307–338.

75. See Louis Brillouin, *Science and Information Theory*, 2nd ed. (New York: Academic Press, 1962), pp. 152–183, esp. p. 168.

76. On phenomenotechnics, see Gaston Bachelard, *La Formation de l'Esprit Scientifique. Contribution à une Psychanalyse de la Connaissance Objective* (Paris: Vrin, 1938), p. 61; Gaston Bachelard, *The New Scientific Spirit*, trans. A. Goldhammer (Boston: Beacon Press, 1984), pp. 3–13; A. Grieder, "Gaston Bachelard: 'Phenomenologue' of Modern Science," *Journal of the British Society for Phenomenology* 17 (1986): 107–122. On embedding and disembedding, see Anthony Giddens, *The Consequences of Modernity* (Cambridge: Polity, 1990).

77. Lacan, *Seminar II*, p. 238.

78. Jacques Derrida, *Given Time: 1. Counterfeit Money* (1991), trans. Peggy Kamuf (Chicago and London: University of Chicago Press, 1992), p. 27.

79. Ibid., pp. 37–38.

80. Ibid., p. 76.

81. See also Jacques T. Godbout in collaboration with Alain Caillé, *L'Esprit du Don* (Paris: Editions La Découverte, 1992), pp. 175ff; François Dosse, *L'Empire du Sens: L'Humanisation des sciences humaines* (Paris: La Découverte, 1995), pp. 151–159; and Maurice Godelier, *L'énigme du don* (Paris: Fayard, 1996).

82. Lévi-Strauss, cited in Borch-Jacobsen, *Lacan: The Absolute Master*, p. 266.

83. Marcel Mauss, *The Gift: Forms and Functions of Exchange in Archaic Societies* (1925), trans. Ian Cunnison, introduction by E. E. Evans-Pritchard, reprinted with corrections (London: Routledge and Kegan Paul, 1969), p. 20, translation modified; see Derrida, *Given Time*, p. 25.

84. Fernand Braudel, *Civilization and Capitalism, 15th–18th Century. Volume II: The Wheels of Commerce* (1979), trans. Siân Reynolds (London: Collins/New York: Harper and Row, 1982), pp. 223ff.

85. Braudel, *The Wheels of Commerce*, p. 226.

86. Ibid., p. 227.

87. Ibid., pp. 228–229.

88. Ibid., p. 229.

89. Ibid., p. 230.

90. On barter, see Caroline Humphrey and Stephen Hugh-Jones, eds., *Barter, Exchange, and Value: An Anthropological Approach* (Cambridge: Cambridge University Press, 1992), especially the Editors' Introduction, pp. 1–20. See also Marshall Sahlins, *Stone Age Economics* (Chicago: Aldine Atherton, 1972) and Nicholas Thomas, *Entangled Objects: Exchange, Material Culture, and Colonialism in the Pacific* (Cambridge, Mass.: Harvard University Press, 1991).

91. Marilyn Strathern, *The Gender of the Gift: Problems with Women and Problems with Society in Melanesia* (Berkeley: University of California Press, 1988), p. 314.

92. The historical development of theories of sexuality from a complementary to a supplementary model is traced in Thomas Laqueur, *Making Sex: Body and Gender from the Greeks to Freud* (Cambridge, Mass.: Harvard University Press, 1990).

93. Jacques Derrida, *Of Grammatology*, trans. with introduction by Gayatri Spivak (Baltimore: Johns Hopkins University Press, 1976).

94. Freud, "From the History of an Infantile Neurosis" (1914/1918), *SE* XVII, 81.

95. See Klein, "The Importance of Symbol-Formation in the Development of the Ego" (1930), in *The Writings of Melanie Klein*, under the general editorship of Roger Money-Kyrle, in collaboration with Betty Joseph, Edna O'Shaughnessy, and Hanna Segal, 4 vols. (London: The Hogarth Press and the Institute of Psycho-Analysis, 1975), vol. I, pp. 219–232; Hanna Segal, "Notes on Symbol-Formation," *International Journal of Psycho-Analysis* 38 (1957): 391–397.

96. Freud, *On Dreams, SE* V, 640.

97. See my essay "What the Psychoanalyst Does with Words: Austin, Lacan, and the Speech Act of Psychoanalysis," in Forrester, *The Seductions of Psychoanalysis: Freud, Lacan, and Derrida* (Cambridge: Cambridge University Press, 1990), pp. 141–167.

98. *E* 322/106, 'Function and Field."

99. On the analogy between money and speech, see the rich work of Marc Shell, *Money, Language, and Thought: Literary and Philosophical Economies from the Medieval to the Modern Era* (Berkeley, Los Angeles, and London: University of California Press, 1982).

100. *Myth* 25/422.

101. *E* 172 (Engl.), "The Freudian Thing."

102. See the incisive Mikkel Borch-Jacobsen, *Lacan: Le maître absolu* (Paris: Flammarion, 1990), pp. 54–60.

103. *E* 126 (Engl.), "The Freudian Thing."

104. See my "Austin, Lacan, et les Actes de Parole en Psychanalyse," *Psychanalyse à l'Université* 10 (1985): 349–367, and the fuller version, "What the Psychoanalyst Does with Words: Austin, Lacan, and the Speech Acts of Psychoanalysis," in Forrester, *The Seductions of Psychoanalysis*, pp. 141–167.

105. *E* 454, "La Psychanalyse et son Enseignement" (1957).

106. Thomas Crump, *The Phenomenon of Money* (London: Routledge and Kegan Paul, 1981), p. 82.

107. Georg Simmel, *The Philosophy of Money*, ed. David Frisby, trans. Tom Bottomore and David Frisby from a first draft by Kaethe Mengelberg, second enlarged edition (London and New York: Routledge, 1990), pp. 510–511. See also p. 169, where Simmel emphasizes that money does not *have* a function, but *is* a function.

108. Karl Marx, *Grundrisse: Foundations of the Critique of Political Economy (Rough Draft)*, trans. with foreword by Martin Nicolaus (Harmondsworth: Penguin, 1973), pp. 165–166.

109. See H. D. Macleod, *The Principles of Economical Philosophy* (London, 1872), 2nd ed.

110. See Stephen Heath, "Notes on Suture," *Screen* 18:4 (1977/78): 48–76.

111. Marx, *Grundrisse*, p. 163.

112. *Timon of Athens*, act 4, scene 3.

113. *E* 692/287, "La signification du phallus."

114. J. M. Keynes, "The General Theory of Employment," *Quarterly Journal of Economics* (February 1937): 215–216, quoted in S. Herbert Frankel, *Money: Two Philosophies* (Oxford: Basil Blackwell, 1977), p. 59.

115. *E* 207 (Engl.), "Possible Treatment."

116. Crump, *The Phenomenon of Money*, p. 91.

117. Lacan, *Séminaire IV*, 30 January 1957, *Bulletin de Psychologie* 10 (1956–57): 742. See the variant in Jacques Lacan, *Le Séminaire. Livre IV. La Relation d'Objet. 1956–1957* (Paris: Seuil, 1994), pp. 153–154.

118. Freud, "On Beginning the Treatment," *SE* XII, 132.

119. Ferenczi, "The Elasticity of Psycho-analytic Technique" (1928), in Sándor Ferenczi, *Final Contributions to the Problems and Methods of Psychoanalysis*, ed. Michael Balint, trans. Eric Mosbacher et al. (London: Hogarth Press and the Institute of Psycho-analysis, 1955), p. 93.

120. Lacan, "Le Séminaire sur 'La Lettre Volée,'" *E* 36.

121. Lacan, *Seminar II*, p. 204; *Le Séminaire. Livre II. Le Moi dans la Théorie*

*de Freud et dans la Technique de la Psychanalyse. 1954–1955* (Paris: Seuil, 1978), p. 239.

122. *FF,* 16 January 1898, p. 294.

123. The dream analysis that Freud published stopped short of revealing this central question of debt to Breuer, which was probably the topic of Freud's conversation with his friend Königstein; Freud did indicate that the question of payment of analytic fees was involved. Jung insisted that the details of this conversation were necessary for understanding the dream and said as much to Freud, implicitly reproving him for not revealing it. This disciple certainly knew when the question of debts was being raised. See my essay "Dream Readers" in Forrester, *Dispatches from the Freud Wars: Psychoanalysis and Its Passions* (Cambridge, Mass.: Harvard University Press, 1997), chap. 4, esp. pp. 173–174.

# ACKNOWLEDGMENTS

How, I wondered, some twenty years ago, does one research a topic like lying, so ubiquitous a practice yet so flimsy in its conceptual outline? At a very early point in my rummaging around in libraries, I discovered the work of a genius: the Catalogue des Matières in the Bibliothèque Nationale in Paris. This anonymous librarian, who obviously knew what was in the texts, had collated the most extraordinary range of interesting works under the rubric of "Mensonge." My project was begun well before keywords had become widespread in libraries and databases, so it was a great boon to discover in this case that an intelligent human being had done the work that computers are now supposed to do more efficiently and comprehensively. Like that most eminent of contemporary students of the everyday, Nicholson Baker, who has been keeping a close eye on the loss of intellectual patrimony that has been quietly accompanying the marvels and miracles of the computerization of libraries, I know that it is not yet plain for all to see that computers can do as good a job of ground-clearing data collation as the humans who formerly worked in our great libraries, so I remain profoundly and knowingly indebted to that exemplary librarian. Among the works that he or she allowed me to find was Alexander Koyré's essay "Refléxions sur le mensonge," a rarity virtually undiscoverable until it was republished in 1996, in elegant booklet form, by Editions Allia in Paris. Here is the second lesson for the scholar: alongside the debt to the librarian is the recognition that one's own secret discoveries and enthusiasms are nearly always shared.

A first version of "Truth Games," the opening essay, was presented, at Anthony Giddens' invitation, to the Social and Political Sciences Seminar, Cambridge University, in March 1979, under the title "Lying on the Couch." Various revised versions, all with considerable reworking, were delivered to the British Society for Philosophy of Science in March 1988, thanks to an invitation from Michael Redhead; to the University of Kent Seminar on Science and Society in March 1988, thanks to an invitation from Crosbie Smith; and to the Architectural Association, London, in May 1988, thanks to an invitation from Mark Cousins; a version was eventually published as "Lying on the Couch" in Hilary Lawson and Lisa Appignanesi, eds., *Dismantling Truth* (London: Weidenfeld and Nicholson, 1989). The present essay is considerably longer than those earlier versions.

An early version of the second essay, "Gift, Money, and Debt," was originally commissioned by Conrad Stein for a conference entitled "Lacan Lecteur de Freud," organized by the Association d'Etudes Freudiennes, September 20–22, 1991, in Paris. A French version of the paper was published in *Etudes Freudiennes* 33 (April 1992): 89–124, and an English version in *Return of the "French Freud": Freud, Lacan, and Beyond*, ed. Todd Dufresne (New York and London: Routledge, 1997), pp. 67–89. The considerably revised and retranslated version published here includes material from a paper entitled "What Are the Consequences of Drawing an Analogy between Speech and Money?" presented to the European Foundation for Psychoanalysis Congress on "The Subject of the Unconscious and Language(s)," generously hosted by Cormac Gallagher in Dublin, Ireland, November 13–15, 1992. Subsequent to the writing of those two papers, I came across Derrida's acute essay *Donner le Temps (Given Time)* of 1991, which addresses so many of the themes that I raise in this essay; its influence has greatly improved the argument.

204

# INDEX

205

placebo and placebo effect, 59–67, 80; definitions, 60, 62; efficacy of, 62–65; and power of mind over body, 76
Plato, 8, 27–28, 91, 179
poet, as liar, 27–28. *See also* fiction
Poincaré, Henri, 38, 41, 42, 146
poker, 49, 179
Polanyi, Karl, 153
politeness and lying, 21
polygraph, 68–69
Popper, Karl, 9, 41, 43
potlatch, 144
Priscillianist heresy, 13, 14, 17
promise, x, 33, 67, 99, 142–143, 151
propositional definition of truth, 38
Proust, Marcel, 21, 22, 23, 26–27, 31–32, 78
*pseudologia fantastica*, 88, 102
psychoanalysis: akin to ethnomethodology, 58; attitude to lying of, 69–70; confidentiality of, 102–107; honesty of analyst in, 93; reality in, 70, 98, 99–101; psychoanalytic model of sexuality, 157–158

Rabelais, François, 129
Ramsey, Frank, 43
reliability of human beings as sources, 53
resistance, 76–77
responsibility, and speech, 140
reversibility in physics, 145–146
Rhyne, Ten, 25
Rousseau, Jean-Jacques, 176
Rushdie, Salman, 101
Russell, Bertrand, 41, 42, 45, 74, 91
Russell's Paradox, 43

Sacks, Harvey, 37–38
Sainsbury, R. M., 41–44
Sainte-Beuve, Charles Augustin, 20
Sartre, Jean-Paul, 8, 16, 96, 97
schizophrenia, 45
science: Augustinian vs. Manichean sciences, 50–52, 53, 69; and horror of deception, 67, 74; as escape, 11–12, 52–53; subject of, 10, 39–40
sciences, opposing ideologies of, 36, 76
scientism, 2–4, 35, 146, 182
Searle, John, 151
secret, society of the, 17
Segal, Hanna, 158
self-deception, 96
sexual relations, barter model of, 157
Shakespeare, William, 19, 20–21, 57
Shapin, Steven, 53
Siegfried, 28
silver, 165
Simmel, Georg, 151, 162
simulation: by computers, 51; and dissimulation, 9–10, 17, 19, 56, 82; in experiments, 54; hysteria as, 68
sincerity, 21, 31
society, dependence of on lying, 20–21
Socrates, 179
speech: and debt, 136, 139–140, 144; founding, 159, 161; full and empty, 141–142; and fundamental rule of analysis, 70–71; idle, 48, 138; and lies, 12, 19; and metaphor of effaced coin, 137–145; and truth, 39
Spiro, Howard, 63–65
Steinbeck, John, *The Grapes of Wrath*, 135
Stevenson, Adlai, 37
Stevenson, Robert Louis, 21
Strathern, Marilyn, 156
Swift, Jonathan, 22–23, 82
Sydenham, Thomas, 68
Symbolic, the, 113, 135–139, 144, 150, 159, 165, 169

*Tarasoff* case, 105–107
Tarski, Alfred, 43
thermodynamics and reversibility, 145–146
Thorndike, Sybil, 24
Tinbergen, N., 141
transgression, pleasure in, 1–2